Time In The Sun

A Record of an Incredible Spiritual Journey

Jill Welch

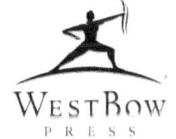

WESTBOW
PRESS

WestBow Press books may be ordered through booksellers or by contacting:

WestBow Press
A Division of Thomas Nelson
1663 Liberty Drive
Bloomington, IN 47403
www.westbowpress.com
1-(866) 928-1240

Because of the dynamic nature of the Internet, any Web addresses or
links contained in this book may have changed since publication and
may no longer be valid. The views expressed in this work are solely those
of the author and do not necessarily reflect the views of the publisher,
and the publisher hereby disclaims any responsibility for them.

ISBN: 978-1-4497-0313-4 (sc)
ISBN: 978-1-4497-0314-1 (e)

Library of Congress Control Number: 2010929965

Unless otherwise indicated, Scripture is taken from the HOLY BIBLE,
NEW INTERNATIONAL VERSION®. NIV®. Copyright © 1973,
1978, 1984 by International Bible Society. Used by permission of
Zondervan. All rights reserved.

For more information visit www.realministries.org

Printed in the United States of America

WestBow Press rev. date: 7/30/2010

To my husband
…with you, I am free to be me.

Contents

Introduction
The Gang

*I*n 1994, I moved to Music City, USA. At the time, the white pages in Nashville were said to be growing by a quarter of an inch each year. Among the immigrants were, of course, the proverbial "busloads" of hopeful singer/ songwriters. As evolution would have it, I became one of the inductees of an infamous group of "busload" girls. This was a group that I had decisively stayed away from for years, arrogantly insistent upon holding firm to my individuality and my illusion of being an artsy elitist.

I considered myself worthy of staying above the fray of such an assembly of women. One by one, though, these girls became an irresistible safety net of interlaced arms underneath a razor-sharp tightrope upon which my feet bled. Eventually, I became one of the "fallen." Christened by an outsider looking in, we went down in Music City history dubbed, "The Gang."

It is phenomenal, yet not surprising in the least to me, that just when I finally got the long-anticipated prompting in my gut to write my story in book form, The Gang takes the stage again. Recently I sat down to attempt to create an ad for a friend's magazine using Adobe Illustrator. I hadn't used the program in a while. So, in playing around in it, perhaps providentially, a design took shape. I had created what looked like a book cover to me. Then I heard it in my spirit, "It's time." A week later, Cynthia, the social butterfly and chief coordinating ringleader of The Gang, emailed a page full of Maxine jokes to the girls of The Gang. I hit "Reply All" and simply typed, "Hey gals! How is everyone?" From there, emails began flying.

It seems as if this happens every year. Someone inevitably suggests some sort of reunion. Everyone begins to draw up their pipe-dream plans of jetting off together to this or that island for a week of pilfering a native community of its very poise. But as inevitably as the creative juices flow in, they quickly flow out and fade to black. This year something feels different, and at this point there are twenty-one and counting girls in this spamorama! I had no idea! My personal circle of friends from The Gang consisted of about ten women. When you begin to add the "Well, I would have never known her if it hadn't been for her" peripherals, it turns out the group was rather large!

Anyway, enough about them. Let's talk about me. This is my story after all. In 1997, out of a deliriously self-absorbed stupor, I let a dreadfully underdeveloped, independently produced record loose from my affirmation-starved hands. It served as an expensive business card that landed me a legitimate publishing deal and a handful of adequate, at best, record deal offers. However, after spending almost a decade in Nashville, and despite countless "holds," I never sold one stinkin' song! I never got to the point of actually "inking" any of the near record deals that flaunted themselves just above reach, like the taunting toys of a crib mobile. I was the baby, too unfocused and uncoordinated to grab one.

I would eventually leave town, unsung. However, one Sunday morning not long before I left, I was seated among the congregation at my home church of several years, before the great Christ Church Choir of Nashville. They were belting out the old hymn "Blessed Assurance," with its familiar refrain: "This is my story, this is my song." As one pastor would later put it, "Jill, your story is your song." As I listened to the choir, the epiphany rose up in me and I shouted inside my own head and heart, "This is my story! *This* is my song!"

My Song

Ten years ago, in a single room in Nashville's Baptist Hospital, I was waking up from the anesthesia when I finally registered the foggy outline of my surgeon's face hanging in mid air over my own. I smiled as I watched words like "tumor" and "chemotherapy" and "radiation" come tumbling, in hazy slow motion, out of his hovering mouth and into my life. As the words translated into some level of reality in my psyche, I turned to find my mother, who was the poster child of tough, non-crying Texas women, with tears streaming down her cheeks. My mouth took it upon itself to open up and tenaciously state, "We have to have faith!" Instantly following that statement, my eyes shut themselves, and we all went back into the safety of the drug-induced dreamland from which we had just mistakenly emerged. It was a supernatural weirdness, the way I fainted back out like that, almost as if I was in control.

I don't know how many hours went by before I woke up again, but when I did I found Stacy, my precious younger sister, sitting in my space and staring me down. I was shocked to see her there. A nurse came into the room, and though I don't remember what all she said, she was like a human angel. She told us she was praying for us all. Then she asked my mother to step out of the room. The minute they closed the door, Stacy leaned in and whispered "OK! What is really going on? I just need to know if Mom has blown this out of proportion or what."

I said something like, "Yeah! OK! Uh well, let's just get the nurse or doctor in here and ask them by ourselves." She said something like, "Yeah, that's a good plan. But we'll have to do it soon, because Rona and Granny just ran to get coffee, and they'll be back any minute." Rona is my older sister, and Stacy must have felt that the less people involved in our covert operation the better.

Rona and Granny? Why is everyone here? I wondered. I was again regaining awareness of my sudden, unwanted reality. Stacy and I had a connection that rarely needed words. So, I was innately trusting that I completely understood where she was coming from. I was even more shocked when it soaked in that they had all actually flown out to Nashville in one afternoon while I was sleeping off the sedation. The entire situation felt as if it was completely out of control. All I could think about now was how this was going to be presented—or, God forbid, how it had already been presented—to my 14-year-old son. My mind was racing. I was desperately trying to sober up and shake the drugs. *But wait,* I thought. *I was here. I heard what the doctor said! Mom isn't making anything up or exaggerating ... is she? What in the world is happening here?*

We never managed to pull off the feat of cornering a nurse or doctor. There was no time for that. I was starving and miserable on every level, and ready to run. I started demanding Kentucky Fried Chicken mashed potatoes and a ride home. Before leaving, I made a less than graceful announcement that I would be the one to tell my son, Slone, what was going on. I wanted to make sure it didn't get conveyed like some scene out of *Terms of Endearment.* This was not a big deal. I had been coherent enough during the surgeon's explanation to understand that he had simply found some little borderline malignant tumor. They cut it out and sent it off for tests. Not a big deal. *What a waste of airfare!* I thought, but I wasn't going to be rude enough to say it.

I was in physical pain and irritated to my very core. I was a completely ungrateful crab and did not care one bit about the feelings of these women who had come rushing to my side to support, comfort, and help me. More than all that, though, they were there to get a grip on their own answers about what in the world was happening, and justifiably so. We'd been through so much. My father had been killed in a car accident, and years later my younger brother was also killed in a car accident. My mother had lost both a spouse and a child, which have to be the hardest losses anyone can survive.

My mother was two months pregnant with me the day of my father's accident. Upon arrival at the hospital where they had rushed my father, my mother began to have symptoms she could not ignore. She was examined by a doctor. With a very cold and harsh bedside manner, he informed her that I was dead. He explained that she would pass the fetus soon. However, that never happened and she soon realized she had not lost me. I had somehow survived her shock and grief. I was there with her, inside the womb, through even her private moments of mourning. I believe I was born with a burden for her. How she is still functional is nothing short of miraculous heroism to me. To say the least, we women have some valid control issues that stem from a love and a fear that runs deeper than the bottom of our hearts.

After situating myself in the bed with the mashed potatoes, I called my son in. He must have at least wondered about the sudden meeting of the matriarchs that was taking place in our apartment living room. He knew that I'd gone in for a "minor" procedure. He came in wearing his usual basketball garb and smelly socks. He made a nosedive for the pillow next to me, as if I wasn't in the least bit of pain from the day's surgery. I was a game-face pro, and I had mine on and locked. We went through a routine line of interrogation.

"Homework?"

"No."

"Yeah right."

"Papers to sign?"

"Nope."

"Mmm hmmm."

"Well, look, this is what happened today. The doctors found a …uh…," I swallowed hard, and then I made a critical error. I locked on, for one split-second too long, to those little brown eyes. I accidentally converged with my own flesh and blood in him – the offspring of the raging river of my very own life. I was suddenly in touch with the power of mortality, and life itself seemed an incomprehensible concept. I could feel the gasp inside, and without warning I burst into a scene of weeping that put Debra Winger and Shirley MacLaine to shame. It was embarrassing, actually, but against my will it continued, because my crying resulted in physical pain, which caused an even louder outburst. I could not seem to grab on and shut it down.

The matriarchs came running. Granny squatted to the floor by my side. Rona and Mom crawled onto the bed with Slone. Then Stacy entered the room, like Joan of Arc breaking through a cloud of war-zone chaos. I could see she was carrying her tiny silver vessel of anointing oil. On the inside, I was rolling my eyes and thinking, *Oh, no. Here she comes with that!* In reality, at that moment I would have let her wipe chicken livers all over me if it would cure anything.

I need to freeze this frame and rabbit trail for a bit. During the few years leading up to this point, I had been on a quest to figure out what I personally believed about God, whether I believed in a "god" at all. The idea of such a quest had been tapping me on the shoulder since I was in my early twenties. Once I'd become an adult, the childhood flannel-board pictures of Jesus knocking on the door of someone's shiny little red heart no longer had enough muscle to keep me reeled in. But who had time to figure all that "heaven and hell" stuff out? I was busy trying to survive life on earth!

Sometime around my 30th birthday, a few things turned me toward the face of that tapping. One was a liberal-minded, world-traveled atheist I was sleeping with for the moment. He was sometimes appalled by my "Southern mindset," as he called it. He suggested that the reason I constantly fell back on Christianity was because I had never known anything else. It was my "back yard," and I had never been out of my back yard, he explained.

Out of pride and my know-it-all character, I would attempt to state my case for Christianity. The more I defended it, the more I sounded like an idiot. I didn't care about being righteous, but I did, by God, care about being right! I hated looking like a fool. There is one thing I've learned though. You can rarely be right when you are uneducated. The truth was that I didn't really know much of anything about anything. I woke up one day after graduating from high school and realized I'd just let twelve years of completely free education go right in one ear and out the other! So I did the only thing an ignorant fool could do. I quickly became an obsessive studier to try and catch up. Now I needed to apply myself in the same way and study religion.

I had gone out with another guy who was one of those turquoise-wearing, soul-seeking, peace-loving kinds of guys. He was a studier too, and he had a countenance that I very much envied. He was not a Christian and didn't have any evident intentions of becoming one, but he was studying Greek and Hebrew in order to read the original biblical transcripts. I called him up and explained my quest. He loaded an entire box up with books on any and every kind of religion you could imagine and lent them to me. He threw in *Jonathan Livingston Seagull* as a bonus.

I pored over these and other books for about a year. I got kicked out of the library on occasion. I also continued poking around in the Bible and reading the mind-honing, circular sub references of C.S. Lewis' *Mere Christianity*. The guy knows how to cover a subject! I had been into *Science of Mind* magazine for several years.

Some friends and I had also been referring Thomas Moore and Deepak Chopra books to each other. If nothing else, the vitally important gift of childlike wonder had been revived in me through all this reading. Then one night at the dinner table, I was trying to discuss an A&E special I had seen on the life of Esther of the Bible. My son stopped me short of finishing, explaining that he had studied this same story in school and that I had the ending wrong. Esther had turned the king into a bullfrog.

I laughed, but then it struck me that he'd been studying something in Greek mythology that at least somewhat paralleled the story of Esther. We had recently gone to see the animated movie *Hercules*. Hercules had a mortal mother and an immortal father. *It's all nonsense!* I thought. I had read the ancient stories that parallel the stories of Adam and Eve, Noah, and other biblical accounts. These stories would take the most bizarre and sometimes entertaining twists and turns from the biblical versions. I compared the timelines of the writings to see which came first, but it proved to be a chicken vs. the egg ordeal. I was getting sick of this silly chase.

To top off the frustration of it all, the more ridiculous it all looked to me, the deeper into Christianity my family back home was getting. It seemed they had all decided to chuck their drugs of choice and stuff Christianity into their pipes. They seemed to be sucking on this stuff as if their lives depended on it, and I was beginning to feel sorry for them. They seemed a bit pathetic with it all, and I was feeling humiliated on their behalf. I remember spilling some sort of Buddhist-ish rambling over the phone to one of them. She, whichever one it was, told me the devil had gotten hold of me. I looked at my atheist sidekick and started sarcastically mocking danger as I re-mouthed her words to him while making little devil horns on my head with my fingers.

Speak of the Devil

*I*t's funny how stubbornly sarcastic I could be about all this. Not long before the atheist had come along, I had an experience with a group of presumably mature, professional, level-headed adults who had somehow gotten caught up in experimenting with a Ouija board. They kept asking me to try it with them. I wasn't afraid of the creepy-crawly mystical edge. I was afraid of my lack of tact, which would inevitably hurt someone's feelings when I made it evident how asinine I thought it was for anyone to be wasting their time on this. There was, I admit, a bit of that Southern mindset telling me that it was somehow my Christian duty to save them all from it before they wound up on the shadowy dark side. God forbid, we'd have to pull one of them out of a static-filled TV screen eventually. I would have to do this gently, though, careful not to offend.

One of them called one night and once again, begged me to join in, because no one else was available to come out and play that night. I finally caved in and went. We each poured ourselves a glass of wine, brought this thing out, and set it up on a small table between us. After a series of simple and somewhat childish questions and a slowly sipped half glass of wine, I was suddenly bowled over by the entrance of a clearly tangible "spirit" in the room. My analytical brain went into hyper mode. *Now how do I know there is a "spirit" in here? Why am I suddenly so convinced?* I was coolly thinking, as I sat back, pointer and thumb resting on chin—suppressing fear. One clue was that when this "spirit" suddenly entered the room, we both simultaneously turned to look at the exact same spot in the room. There was no reason to assume this "spirit" was in one or another particular part of the room. I was challenged by this phenomenon, to say the least. The spirit had a name. He had a gender, and he had a distinct personality. He just didn't have skin.

More and more people were getting involved in this practice. There was another Christian involved, and she approached me at a party one night. She asked me about my feelings on it, and I started giving her stock Christian lip service: "Oh yes. I know. I've been praying about it, and I don't think it is something we should be messing with." My analytical side was hooked, though. I was too engrossed in investigating it to worry much about any impending spiritual danger. The longer this went on, the more I was reeling about the paranormal. This thing was telling us things about people that would turn out to be true or that would later happen. It was incredible.

I was still meticulously skeptical, though. I would go back and forth about whether this was all in our heads. I would become convinced that we were simply stirring this up in one another and causing ourselves to believe something we wanted to believe. It was stimulating and exciting. Then one day I was writing a letter to a guy I had started dating. He wanted to "get serious" much sooner than I wanted. The last line of the letter read, "I am dancing as fast as I can." The minute I signed my name and put the pen down, the phone rang, and I was invited to come join the group for another session that was already in progress. A new spirit had introduced itself, and they wanted me to come check it out.

I stopped by Burger King on the way over and got food. When I arrived, there were four people on the board. There wasn't really room for me, and I wanted to eat. I sat on the couch and listened in as I ate. It didn't seem to me that any new spirit was present at the moment. Then I said, "Hey, ask it if I can ask questions from over here." I was pretty cynical and worn out by the little game that day. They asked, and it said, "Y-e-s." With a testing attitude I asked, "OK—what do I do about this relationship I've gotten myself into?" The group turned to the board, and they all again, started in on the juvenile ritual of spelling out loud. "D(slide)… A(slide)…N (slide)…C (slide)…E (stop)." They looked up at me with puzzled frowns.

"You have got to be kidding me!" I said. That was it for me. I was convinced, and I am to this day convinced. I no longer had any doubts about the existence of a very real realm, separate and outside of us. These things simply could not just be in our heads. That group knew nothing about my letter to my boyfriend, and it was not possible in the least that this was a coincidence.

A few weeks later, I got a phone call from one member of the group. It was late at night. She was with the group, and she was frantic. I could hear the group murmuring in the background, and it was clear something was wrong. She explained that something terribly dark had just happened. She pleaded with me to get rid of anything in my house that was connected in any way with this thing we'd all been messing with. She said they would explain later what had happened.

I never got much of an explanation though, because once the situation of that night subsided, no one ever wanted to talk in depth about it again. Some claimed they had literal struggles with getting a presence of evil out of their houses and even out of their very bodies. These were the same people who for months had been adamantly defending the innocence and value of this practice.

One day months later, the atheist and I were headed somewhere when he realized he missed his turn. He drove into the parking lot of a temple to turn around. I began to feel a strange tension and feeling of being pulled into a place I didn't want to be. It quickly got heavier and heavier. The air seemed thick and luring. He tried several ways to turn the car around in this parking lot, but nothing worked.

Once he finally got the car free and back out on the street, he shouted "Damn! That was evil! There was something evil in there!"

I perked up. "Oh my gosh! You recognized it? Did you hear what you just said?" I asked.

"Well," he stammered, "I... I do believe there are ... energy fields... uh, you know, magnetic, negative energy fields out... out there."

I had to point it out. "But, you actually used the word 'evil'. What does that mean to you?" I asked. I could tell it was useless to push him on the subject, so I dropped it.

Even after the atheist was long gone, I eventually renounced the title "Christian," implementing the popular label "spiritual" instead. I put my personal quest to bed in one fell swoop. I had several of the books I'd been studying strewn out all over the kitchen table. In frustration I put down the one I had in my hand and leaned back in the chair. I looked up at the ceiling and said something I now wish I had said years before.

"OK! Enough of this! I don't know who you are or *if* you are. I don't know if you are Buddha or Mohammad or a committee of ten thousand Martians—and I really don't care which one. I just want to know the TRUTH!" I shouted. "So, I'm asking you, whoever or whatever you are, to reveal yourself to me. The way I figure it is that if I ask that and you don't reveal yourself then there is no God. If there is a God who will not answer this question for me, then this game is too unfair to play, and I am not ever going to worry about this again!" I walked away with a "So, knock yourself out. I'll be waiting!" attitude. I loaded the box up with the books and gave it back to my friend, returned books to the library, and shelved the ones I owned.

By then, Slone had gotten "plugged in," as they called it, to a Baptist youth group. Even though I was no longer a "Christian," I was still attending Christ Church. I had originally chosen Christ Church because it was across the street from our apartment. I don't know why I kept going to church, but Sunday after Sunday, I would show up there a disheveled, miserable mess.

I always sat up in the balcony where no one would bother me. It happened to be across the aisle from where Naomi, Wynonna, and occasionally, Ashley Judd sat. I felt hidden up there, overshadowed by their fame. Sometimes they would come up there, inside the church with their big hair and big personas, attempting to hide behind big sunglasses, and I wished I could get away with that, to hide my hangovers – and my whole self.

I began noticing that I could not escape the word "baptism." I could not get away from this word. It was popping up everywhere. Slone had been baptized not long before. He invited me to his church to witness his baptism. To me, witnessing it was a little like watching a really important fifth-grade play. I really didn't understand baptism but I was inspired by Slone's passion and sincerity about it. I got offended though, because his pastor actually instructed his congregation to raise their hands in the air during a worship song. I'd been around these hand-raising people in a charismatic church in Amarillo, Texas that I attended with Stacy. It freaked me out. I found it desperate and silly. There were a few of these types at Christ Church, but I didn't notice them so much from the balcony.

It seemed to be more and more frequent that this word, baptism, would show up. Then one day, out of the blue, my mother called me. Completely out of character, she said, "Jill, for some reason I feel like I am supposed to talk to you about baptism." I almost fell in the floor. I kept my cool, though, afraid that by the time I hung up, I'd have committed to attend some tent revival somewhere. When I got off the phone I sat in silence for a moment, contending with the undeniable confirmation in what had just happened.

I had to admit that every time I went from reading any spiritual or religious material to reading the Bible, I would clearly notice a significant difference. The Bible kept ringing true to me. It felt right. It felt native to something in me, but I just kept chalking that up to my atheist friend's "back yard" theory. However, I decided to see what the Bible had to say about baptism. I looked up the word in a concordance and read any and every passage that mentioned baptism, baptize, or Baptist.

When I finished this word study, I felt that I had some level of innate understanding of baptism but not a tangible understanding, almost as if someone had verbally taught me how to paint without ever showing me a canvas or brush. It was enough, though, and I knew I had to do this.

Although I wasn't ready to fully admit it, Christianity was stirring and connecting inside me. With my heels digging in the dirt, I was reluctantly becoming more resolute, which was disappointing because I had become very accustomed to the social acceptance and liberties that came from being free of the taboo associated with the "Christian" label. I made the decision to be baptized in Dallas over Christmas so my family could be a part of it and be so proud of me. I was apparently joining their club, but I was still holding fast to some personal opinions and conditions in this decision.

I began watching a television pastor out of Austin, Texas named Gerald Mann. He was a down-to-earth, rational, wise man, and I liked him. My older sister, Rona, was into Joyce Meyer and T.D. Jakes, the way she'd been into Stevie Nicks and Lindsey Buckingham in the '80s. Stacy had been attending a church that was in the middle of a rather lengthy "move of the Holy Spirit" —whatever that was. My mother was more in the mode of "I didn't write the rules, God did. Here they are. Like it or not, we have to follow them!" And to top it all off my stepmother and Stacy had somehow miraculously managed to get my super indifferent dad to be more serious about God and church than I'd ever seen him be. Even Slone was preaching at me by then.

I got baptized, but anticipating the likes of the story Rona told of her own baptism, I was disappointed when I didn't feel as if I'd become some sort of levitated essence when I came up out of that water. But what was done was done. I had made my official public announcement that I was indeed a Christian. I would never become one of those silver-fish-sticker-toting Christians who apparently didn't have enough of a life to think about anything outside of Christianity, but I was "in" nonetheless.

The fact was that I had finally admitted to myself that the more I studied all those books, the more it seemed clear to me that Christianity had to be the exclusive truth. I was tiring of the belief in "many truths." "What is true for you is not necessarily true for another," people would claim, in that tone that sounded as if they had just stepped out of a three-week stint in a sweat lodge. For me, there was a simple equation that proved that truth is exclusive. The equation is two plus two, which is four for everyone, which consequently excludes three and five and three point nine, nine, nine, etc.

If there is one truth, then all other claims must somehow exist under the umbrella of that one truth. When I would piece it all together like a puzzle, the only amalgamation of all these doctrines and theories that made sense was that Christianity was that umbrella. In that arrangement, I could see that all these other religions teach partial truths along with deceptive doctrine that twists and perverts the authenticity found in the Bible.

A friend uses the analogy of strychnine. It only takes a solution of 2 percent strychnine to kill you. Many of these religions seem to convey 98 percent truth and 2 percent poison. The study of all these religions only served to point me right back to the glaring deduction that this God of the Bible is the one true God. Now, here I was just a few short weeks from my valiant move in and out of the waters of baptism, released from the Baptist Hospital, holding a Styrofoam vat of mashed potatoes and the diagnosis of massive chaos. I had surely picked the wrong god after all!

Joan of Arc

So, back to Joan of Arc and her anointing oil… Stacy stepped up and said, "We need to pray." Now, we were all praying people but not the stand-in-a-circle, holding-hands, and praying-out-loud kind. None of us, that I knew of, were comfortable with praying out loud except Stacy. I remember a time not long before this when Rona called. We needed to pray for someone, and we knew it. She said, "I think we should pray right now about this." I said, "Yes, we should…Let's do that… You go ahead…" There was a pause. "No you…you start, and I'll finish." Then we both laughed realizing how strange it was that we were so tentative about praying out loud together.

At Stacy's prompting, everyone assumed various prayer positions—heads bowed and eyes closed. Stacy rubbed some of the oil on the top of my hands and smoothly rolled into a very relaxed and conversational prayer, knowing just what to say and just what to ask for.

After a few minutes of eloquent beseeching, Mom interrupted her by softly tapping her on the leg. "And…and Stacy, ask Him if …" I don't remember specifically what she was requesting because we all lovingly laughed about it.

Stacy paused for a moment, looked up and said "Well Lord, you heard her."

This time of prayer was a precious experience. This was a moment of harmonized, mutual surrender that we had never captured before. Together we allowed ourselves to be completely vulnerable and at the mercy of this God we all claimed we believed in.

What happened next will be the most difficult thing in this book for me to write about. As I have said so many times before about this, there are simply no words valuable or weighty enough to describe it. But I continue to do my best with what I have to work with—the English language.

I did not tell anyone about this experience for months. I chose not to, because it felt too hard to describe, because I never wanted to give room for any sort of petty human argument about it, and because it was a tremendous reality to contend with. I wasn't sure I was ready to talk about it. Admitting it would force me to face it.

The prayer had ended, and everyone had left the room so I could sleep. I don't remember lying there long when instantly a dire fear came over me. This was a fear so intense it seemed insurmountable, almost as if I would not live through it. It was as if a flock of black vultures swooped in and landed in my emotions and began devouring me from the inside out. Every time I look back on it that is what I involuntarily picture. I had no idea what to do, but I was not about to cause another scene. So I kept my mouth shut and thought for a second.

I hate taking painkillers, but there next to me on the nightstand was the small bottle containing a few Hyrdrocodone pills, prescribed after surgery. Hoping they would knock me out and serve as the quickest way to escape from this horrendous living nightmare, I sat up in the bed and reached for the small bottle and water glass, and quickly took a pill. Then I reached and turned the lamp off. Still sitting up, I immediately turned my body back to center in order to lie back down. In mid turn I was frozen stiff. I could see a translucent and luminescent figure sitting beside me on the bed. It was like the light from a film projector, in that, while you can place your hand into its light stream, it still has a tangible, cone shape. It was clearly a man wearing a white linen robe. His hands were draped over his bending knees, and he was sitting, silent and still, right there beside me. This was not a vision happening inside my head. This was happening in the material, physical realm before my eyes. This was a man on my bed in my bedroom in my apartment in Nashville, Tennessee!

I realized that the darkness and fear that had set in had immediately moved to the distance. This was not out of "spiritual sight," so to speak. I could sense the presence of a terrible, dark, threatening spirit standing near my closet, but there was a knowing in me that it could not even begin to penetrate the power that encircled me. It was as if I was inside an invisible bubble of power. I could see out, but nothing could get in. This man beside me was the epitome and personification of the phrase "at rest."

I could not move, but even if I could have, I would not have been able to turn and look him in the eyes. I inherently knew, without question, that it would be beyond unbearable. Again, there are no words that could begin to touch this level of power. But in the frozen stiffness, I was completely immersed and engulfed in the most concentrated influence and sensation of peace and comfort and safety.

It was a serenity that made me recognize how desperately uneasy, uncomfortable, and unsafe I had been all my life. It was a devastating awakening —devastating in the sense that I had no idea how truly miserable I had been until that moment. I would never again be satisfied to live in that level of misery.

As well as I know when my own mother enters the room, I knew who this was next to me. There was not even a split second of questioning in me about who or what this was. My physical intellect knows and instantly recognizes my mother, and my spiritual intellect knew and instantly recognized my Creator. This was Jesus.

For as many times as I have gone over this experience in my own head, digging deep to analyze it, I am not able to doubt that, for even a second, since it happened ten years ago. I remain willing to discover that I am wrong and that this experience was a byproduct of shock or something along those lines, but I have not found it in me to become convinced of that as of yet. I am telling you that I know that I know this was Jesus.

How this moment waned, I cannot fully recollect, but when it did, for some odd reason I picked up my guitar. I began playing a simple little melody line, and as I was playing it, I seemed to be sending that sound up as a musical prayer. As the sound went up, more of the melodic line would come to me, and I would play it. The melody would bring a peace to my soul, as if it was the answer to the musical prayer. It was an incredible circular thing that was happening. I was offering up this sound, and then more melody was falling down; peace would come, and then I would offer up that sound and so on. I tried to sleep but couldn't. I was on a calm and peaceful high.

All of this happened within a matter of a few minutes. I noticed that my hands were hot, as if they were on fire. I got out of bed and went into the living room. With a tranquil countenance, I said, "I don't know what is going on, but my hands are on fire!" My Granny stood up and said, "Well, put 'em on me!" Granny, I learned later, was a bit of a closet charismatic. I smiled and placed my hands on both of her wonderfully soft cheeks. I was glad to do so. Her sweet face was one of my favorite things in the world!

The first-time euphoria of Hydrocodone finally kicked in, and I fell asleep. My mother, needing to be as close as possible, slept with a blanket and pillow on the floor at the foot of my bed that night. My mother is not an overtly affectionate person. She was never able to say, "I love you" when I was young, but she has her own ways of showing her love. The Lord just recently showed me that her sleeping on the floor that night was one of the purest.

Cancer

The next morning, after some great drug-induced sleep and some food, I was clear-minded and eager to get to the bottom of all of this. Stacy and I devised a plan to get the surgeon on the phone, and we would both listen to him together. She listened in on the phone in Slone's room. I explained to him that I needed to go over everything again.

Stacy and I both had notepads in hand. He began to explain again that he had discovered a Stage III, borderline malignant, ovarian tumor. He explained that there was no chemotherapy or radiation that had proven to be effective for this particular type of tumor. "Borderline malignant" basically meant that these tumors would not be quickly spread by way of blood cells. "However," he added, "the particular type of borderline malignant tumor that you have typically spreads in sheets." In other words, typically where one tumor is found, several others are found in the surrounding area. He explained that he was advised to stop the surgery and not proceed until he received the full tests back from the lab. "That is why I am referring you on to the oncologist. She will help me decide how to proceed," he explained.

I remember thinking, *What exactly is cancer? And what is a tumor? And do you have cancer if you have a tumor, and do you have a tumor if you have cancer?* I finally interrupted him and asked, "OK. But is this actually cancer?" There was the slightest scary pause, and then he answered, "Yes." The word "yes" had never had that effect on me. But then, after another short pause, he added, "Technically, yes."

OK, wait, I thought. *Don't oncologists exclusively deal with cancer?* Was he dancing around the real truth? Was he breaking it to me gently? He assured me they would be able to explain it better once the test results came in. He hoped to have the results in time for our scheduled follow-up appointment. So, it appeared that I had what I started calling "a mild case of cancer." I sat up in the bed after hanging up and began to ask, and test, and feel, to see if the Lord would come in that way again. It was daylight, and that somehow made it seem unlikely, but I tried Him anyway. I sat there but felt nothing. I waited a little longer—still nothing.

There was so much to suddenly sort out. I began to pray my normal, silent-type of praying. Sometimes I had a hard time praying, because when I would try, every filthy thought known to man would show up on the screen of my mind. I would think to myself *Geez! I can't talk to God and think about that at the same time!* But somewhere in my search for ultimate truth I guess I finally had gotten desperate enough to break through all that and pray anyway. I didn't have any trouble this day, and one of the first questions or fears that came to me during my prayer was that I was going to wind up having to leave Nashville and move back to Texas. I hated Texas, and I loved Nashville with a passion.

My sisters and Granny went back, but we got word that Granny had fallen in the airport. She was traveling alone, but some very sweet people had come to her rescue. I felt so bad for her, but it was just another unfortunate incident I couldn't do anything about. I noticed some strange behavior in her, but I assumed she was just in shock like the rest of us. Her fall caused me to be even more concerned.

Mom planned to stay with me, and we went to the follow-up appointment together. I was lying on the examining table in the surgeon's office after he had checked my blood pressure and all of the typical stuff. He was sitting on one of those rolling stools and had rolled over to the counter next to where my mother was seated. He was making those scary, secret notes inside a manila folder. My mom stopped him with her eyes and said, "Look, I need to know what we are really dealing with here."

Anger began filling me up and I thought, *Please don't ask any more questions. Let me ask when I'm ready. I can only soak in so much of this at one time. I haven't even digested the confusing diagnosis I've gotten so far.* I turned just in time to watch him lower his head and say, "She's in trouble." My spirit fell.

He looked at his notes and began explaining again. He had filmed the original surgery. He had even given us a copy of it at the hospital before we left. What a strange parting gift that was! I hadn't had the guts to watch it. Based on the lab results, they decided that I needed to go in for more exploratory surgery and a hysterectomy. He was forced to remove the one ovary already. When I finally did have the guts to watch the film, I saw that he quickly turned the camera off upon discovering the tumor.

The news of the hysterectomy was heart-shattering to me. The reason I had gone in for this routine laparoscopic surgery in the first place was because I had myself convinced that the Lord was about to take care of some long-suffered female trouble and enable me to have children again someday. I had wanted to have more children for years and had not been able to since having Slone. I was dating someone at the time, and there was even some light talk of marriage, but I wanted this in general. I had goals calendared out in my head, and I had always planned on having children again at 35. I had just turned 33. I felt I had no choice, and the second surgery was scheduled two weeks after the first one. I cried my eyes out over this. I sulked. I stewed. I cussed. There was no option but to suck it up and get through all this. So I did.

I don't remember how or when the news of all this was broken to the girls of The Gang, but they could not have rushed quicker or gone more out of their way to support me. I think this "mild case of cancer" diagnosis was as confusing for them as it was for me and my family. Some did research on it. We had a friend who was best friends with the oncologist in New York who had treated both Jackie Onassis and Linda McCartney. He was more than willing to review my case. I hated to be ungrateful, but I couldn't help thinking, *but Jackie O and Linda are both dead.* One of the girls discovered in her research that I had a 50 percent chance of living. In cancer terms, those are more than great odds—but talk about glass half empty or half full! It was truly all in how you looked at it.

Mom was staying with me, and Rona planned to come back to Nashville a couple of days after the surgery. The surgery went well. The doctor said he saw nothing of concern and felt great about the pending results. He told us the lab results would be back in a few days.

I was dying to see my friends. I had not seen them in weeks, and I was realizing more than ever before how dependent I had become on them and how deeply I loved and appreciated them all. Rona offered to drive me to go to lunch with Cassie and Cynthia. They were two of my closest friends from The Gang.

I wanted so badly to do something normal, something that would make the statement that I was done with that little bit of chaos and ready to move on. I was unable to receive any sort of hormone replacement therapy until my medical team had decided for certain that they would not need to use chemotherapy. Being slammed into the wall of menopause and attempting to endure hot flashes was almost unbearable. A wave would hit, and I would feel like I was going to fall to the floor. What a phenomenon these little woolly boogers are! The body and its functions and malfunctions are beyond astounding.

I was expected to tolerate these episodes, but it was staggering how powerfully upsetting they were. Rona, bless her heart, is not the strongest camper in the troop. She is too sensitive and empathetic, and I thought we were never going to make it to this lunch. She was almost begging me to let her turn the car around and take me home, but she also knew how badly I wanted and needed to do this. It was not so great to see the girls. I was in agony, and as much as I tried to fake my way through, it was obvious. Everyone tactfully ate fast and delicately urged me to go home.

When we got home, Mom had this great look of accomplishment written all over her face. She had been on a mission to buy me a Bible. She had this somewhat strange list of criteria for the Bible she wanted to find. She wanted it to be navy blue with silver-lined pages. It had to have thumb tabs, because she correctly assumed I did not know my way around the Bible. And lastly, it had to be an NIV (New International Version) Study Bible. This is a plain-English version that kindly dropped all the confusing thee's and thou's and such, and also included study notes at the bottom of each page with further breakdown and explanation of each scripture.

She proudly described how at the first Christian bookstore she went to, on the first shelf she looked at, the first Bible she saw fit this exact description. She walked right up to it and knew it was the one. She had them engrave my name on the front. She was beaming as she presented it to me. I was terribly preoccupied with the fact that I could not seem to get the reins of my life back into my hands. She sat on the edge of my bed and read scripture to me. I barely recognized it in the moment. What an incredible turnaround this was from our former lives. I didn't even slow down enough to appreciate it.

The surgeon finally called with the results of the lab tests. Waiting on these results was brutal, to say the least. Immediately I noticed that he sounded defeated and sad and apologetic. He explained that the tests had shown that there were tiny tumors covering the back side of the uterus as well as various places in the abdominal cavity. These tumors were being found in adhesions. Mom and I had watched the film and could see that the liver was of concern as well. The greater concern at that point, he explained, was the colon. He insisted that I agree to schedule an emergency surgery as soon as I had recovered enough from the last surgery. He further explained that this surgery would more than likely require a temporary colostomy. He said he was very sorry to have to give me this report and that he was as surprised as I was. The decision was mine, but he sounded as if it was urgent that I agree with this advice. He had scheduled an appointment for me to meet with the oncologist who had been counseling him in the decisions he had to make.

Cassie Berns, a prominent and beloved member of The Gang, was a "soul-connection" for me like no other in that group. Before moving to Nashville, I started hearing a country version of Janis Joplin's "Piece of My Heart" in my head. At the time I had an acoustic trio with my then-husband and our friend Johnny Rose. I begged the guys to let me try it. They both looked at me as if I was crazy and resolutely agreed, "No way!" They finally acquiesced somewhat and let me do an acoustic MTV-style, "unplugged" version. Just before we all moved to Nashville, Faith Hill put out the now famous country version of this song. The guys never properly apologized. I am still waiting.

Cassie's father, the late Bert Berns, wrote that song, among many other hits. I was introduced to Cassie, and mutual friends had told her this story about me. In turn, Cassie told me the story of how she too had begun hearing a country version in her head. She had cut a demo with high expectations of launching her own country record based on covering her father's song.

The demo apparently made the rounds on Music Row and into the hands of Faith Hill's producer. He apparently thought it was a good idea too. I think Cassie is still waiting for an apology herself, but that's her story to tell.

We immediately clicked, and I love that girl like she's a part of me. We both had "tough girl syndrome," and over a couple of glasses of any given alcohol, we could toss our hair back and laugh our way out of any kind of pain. So, I decided she would be the one I would call with the news. Again, not expecting it in the least, I fell apart on the phone, embarrassed myself to death, and quickly hung up.

Cynthia was our mutual best friend. She was also the nurturing one of the bunch. Cynthia was the one you wanted to be around when you were in trouble. She just happened to be in Cassie's office and was there to console her as Cassie put her head down on her desk and cried.

I couldn't understand all this involuntary weeping from all the tough girls. I grew up with and learned from the best, and even I couldn't stop breaking down. I hardly ever cried before this! I prided myself on this fact. Everything was just so out of control. Logic kept telling me this was absolutely no big deal, but then this unruly element just kept permeating the air. It was like a belligerent, wild horse that I wasn't dominant enough to tame.

I continued to pray. I was in an almost constant state of prayer. People from all over the world, it seemed, were sending emails telling us that they were praying for me. The most bizarre on the list was a former lover of Bill Clinton's who had later become a Christian. I don't personally know this woman, and I don't remember now how she made this list. I could at times feel a wave of what I knew was the power of prayer. A few days after this conversation with the surgeon I began to have a dialog with God. I felt convinced that God was telling me that I was ultimately going to die from this. It wasn't going to be any time soon, but that I needed to get my "house in order" and prepare for it.

Because of the scale of the experience of that first night, I was tuned in and believed what I was hearing and sensing. My initial reaction to this was one of pure amazement and wonder. God was the final authority, and I took Him at His word. I opened wide my spiritual arms and felt drenched in awe of the concept. *We are talking about the big transition from here to there,* I'd think. It was mind-boggling and thrilling at first. I was learning that you don't necessarily need to share every detail of your process with the people around you in a situation like this. I found myself needing to stay above the reactions and responses of people and carry the burden of some of it on my own. I wasn't about to share this.

A couple of days of this unadulterated acceptance went by when I began to question God. *But wait. I don't understand this. Why would you take me now?* I thought. *I just completely gave my life to You, and I was really getting close to being ready to "shout it from the mountaintop." So why now?*

My mom sat on the opposite couch and abruptly blurted out the question. "Jill, I need to know. Do you think you are going to die?" She must have been hearing it too. Strangely devoid of almost any emotion, I answered, "Well, since you asked, I think the Lord is telling me that. I don't feel it will be in the next few days or weeks or anything. But, I think He's telling me to get things in order." She slowly lay down on the couch. Looking back I realize that from that moment, she began to wither like a leaf before my eyes. She had been doing so well in recent years. The grief of losing my brother took a toll on her that seemed impossible to overcome on any and every level. She tells the story of how she had to finally get on her knees and fully surrender the loss and my brother to God. She had miraculously been turning a corner—and now this.

A couple of days later, my true feelings hit me. Lying there, I turned to hide my face from whoever might be walking through the living room and began to silently cry and silently cry out. Whether or not it was OK for me to challenge God on such a thing, I wasn't sure. I had an all new level of reverence after the experience I'd had, but I also had an all new level of trust and comfort with Him.

I finally said, "OK, God, I know that You are sovereign and in complete authority and control. I know I don't really have a say in this, but I cannot just open my arms up and accept this without at least saying this: 'I am not ready to go! I just am not. I cannot comprehend the thought of leaving Slone. He is everything in this world to me. I know I have not been a great mother, but I cannot stand the thought of leaving him. There is still so much I want to do with my life. I want to live to be 105. I've never fully realized that, but I'm serious—I really do. So, if it's OK for me to ask this, then I am asking You if I can stay!" I left it at that. The rest, in my understanding, was up to Him.

I had been feeling a tug getting increasingly noticeable, but I was ignoring it. I had been ignoring this for years. Rona was on her way out the door to run some errands for me when, out of some deep-rooted impulse, I said, "Wait. I have to say something!" She stopped. "OK," she said as she sat on the floor near the coffee table. Mom sat up on the couch. "I don't know why but I have to say this. I think all of this somehow has something to do with what I'm about to say." I was so nervous I could hardly talk.

I'd kept my little secrets for so long. This was the one secret, among the others, that I knew I could confess without upsetting the whole world. "I was raped in high school, and I never told anyone about it." A silence visibly landed inside both of them as they stared at me. Mom finally leaned in, and with a rare gentleness about her, she said, "This is not to take away from what you might have gone through, but do you realize that one out of four girls have gone through the same thing?"

I knew the statistics. Hers was low. It was one in three, according to my research. Instead of taking in the gentleness in her tone, I immediately zeroed in on the feeling that I was going to be simply written off as a statistic. I silently said, *See, God? Now what good did that do?* She again assured me that she was not taking lightly what I had said, but in my mind I had been disregarded. Being disregarded by people was a familiar painful pattern in my life, and I simply wasn't going to sit there holding my finger in that socket. I said something like, "Yeah, I don't know why. I just thought I needed to say that." I closed the door on the subject. It was never mentioned again. Rona went to the store, and as usual, life went on.

We received news from back home that Granny had suffered a major stroke. She was unable to speak as a result of it. I watched my mom sit in a chair and stare out the French doors for what seemed like hours. Occasionally she would talk about the tragedy of losing the ability to communicate with her own mother. Granny was our source of tenderness. She and my grandfather—we call him Boompa—provided my only real sense of home. I have deeply dreaded losing them since I was a young girl.

At some point in the midst of all the ongoing upheaval, Rona came in and sat on the edge of my bed. She said, "Listen, we've been talking, and we think it would be best if I took Slone back to Dallas with me. I think we could get him under control, and this way there will be someone there to watch his ball games." This felt like the most blind-siding string of statements I could have ever imagined coming out of her mouth. I was not one who could ever easily state her true feelings, but I was getting more and more irritable. I felt I was being swarmed and suffocated by all of this. I was losing tact.

I got pregnant with Slone in my senior year of high school. His father and I began hanging out with the same group of kids. My first love had recently broken up with me, and I had aimlessly wandered into this new circle of friends. We were the only two within the group who were not dating anyone. So, by default, we became a couple.

I was known for smoking pot, winning tequila shot contests, and writing embarrassing amateur country songs. He was a straight-laced honor student and super-jock. We could not have been more polar opposite. But there we were, available and in the same room. I was well programmed by that time to think that I was some sort of sexual object, and having sex was simply my duty. It was not long before we were sleeping together.

I had toyed with the picket-fence talk of marrying him after graduation, but we both secretly knew that was never going to happen. He was being scouted by the likes of the Toronto Blue Jays, while my mom and I had plans to load up the bad songs and head out to "NashVegas."

I knew I was pregnant even before the nurse called to confirm it. The call obviously sparked an overwhelming sensation, but I was not shocked to find that out because something in me was rapidly and drastically changing. With the confirmation of this fact, I knew that I had miraculously changed overnight.

Before this, I could have cared less if the sun came up the next day. I was suddenly not the same Jill. I was instantly connected to this little invisible life, and it was a transforming experience. No one could discern this, and it wasn't something I was interested in trying to convince people of. They would make their smart-mouthed, judgmental remarks, but I knew and that was all that mattered.

Years went by before I would fully realize that this unborn life represented a gift of pure and untainted love. I had needed that kind of love so badly for so long. I let my whole broken life fall into the well of the matchless love that can only be shared between a mother and a child she cherishes.

In recent years people have lovingly suggested that I watch a movie called *Juno*. They tell me how awesome and adorable this movie is. They say I will identify with it. "Because," they add, "this must have been the way it was for you." I finally watched the movie. While I understand why they came to that conclusion, my experience, for the record, was nothing like that. It is a tragedy to me that so many people find endearing this story of a young girl who is so completely apathetic about the indescribable, immeasurable privilege of delivering a human being into life.

Abortion was not something that would register in me, even for a moment. I had friends who'd had abortions. I didn't have judgmental feelings about that. However, some confided in me, sharing the details of their utter torment over it. It was terribly distressing to me.

I considered adoption but only long enough to know that there was no way I could let this go. This felt like something so special. This was not something I could or wanted to somehow shake off and run from. I immediately embraced having this child with all that was in me.

After Slone was born, one day I was warming bottles of milk on the stove at my grandfather's. I was holding him in my arms and staring into this beautiful child's face. I didn't realize my grandfather had stopped in the door of the kitchen and was watching me. "My God! You love that boy, don't you?" he said in a half whisper. He startled me, and as I turned I could see a look of wonder on his face. I smiled. I knew that he recognized this change in me. It was a great moment between us.

Slone's father and I did marry after high school. We made a noble attempt to make it work, but neither of us was equipped for that level of challenge. I left for good when Slone was 4. I let go of the idea of any real music career for the first few years of Slone's life. I dabbled in playing with bad bar bands but never felt that I was getting anywhere with that. It was a time-consuming way to make a little extra money, but I could do it while Slone was asleep at a babysitter's house.

Slone and I lived in absolute poverty. At the lowest point, in 1985, I was making $3.60 an hour with no child support. There was one period of time in that year when we had nothing to eat for days except a box of dry cereal that I was carefully rationing.

So, when Slone was 8 years old I sat him down and finally said, "Look, right now I make $7 an hour, and you see how we live. It is likely that I will never make much more than this but, I have these songs," I explained. "It would take a sacrifice for both of us. I would have to work during the day and at night, but if we went to Nashville, I might get lucky and pull us out of this." He looked up with a sweet, beaming smile and said what he knew I wanted to hear: "Let's do it, Mom!"

After a few self-consumed years in Nashville and a second failed marriage, I had put Slone through the ringer. My constant prayer had been, "I want to be successful out here, but above anything else, I want to be a good mother." The truth is, I did want that more than anything, but it seems I thought that prayer would work like some magic word. I could be as selfish as I wanted as long as I was saying that. I assumed God would answer this commanding prayer of mine, and with no real effort or action on my part, somehow I would still pull off a "Mother of the Year" miracle.

Anger issues were boiling to the top for Slone from years of my neglect, constant disorder, and lack of stability and structure. Hurt people hurt people, as they say. In my unhealed anger and bitterness I was too often verbally abusive. There were even times over the years when I believe I occasionally crossed the line into what I would consider physical abuse. Sometimes this abuse was accidental or unintentional. In the wildness of unhealed emotions, discipline escalated to physical struggle. In my immaturity and ignorance of how to properly raise a child, I regretfully allowed things to spin out of control.

Slone was beginning to get in trouble at school too often. One night, in a fit of long-suppressed anger, Slone ripped through the dining room, turning over the table and every last chair. I knew it had gotten out of hand and something had to be done. I made the decision to send him to live with his dad. I got on my knees to pray that night for the first time in years.

I recognized that every single thing that I had touched in my life had fallen apart. Slone was the one thing I was determined not to fail, but I had. I pulled the untouched Bible off the bookshelf it had been sitting on for years. I opened up to the book of Proverbs and began to read it. I put Slone on an airplane to his father's and came home as empty inside as I had ever been in my life.

I continued to read Proverbs, but it was about this time that the atheist entered the scene. With Slone gone I had more time and freedom to stay out at night and party. Drinking was becoming an everyday habit for me. There was always a reason to celebrate on Music Row. Someone got a number-one hit. Someone released a record. Someone signed a deal.

I realized that I was drinking by noon some days, and I was getting a little alarmed. During that period, the atheist had appeared and disappeared. My moral bar was lowering by the minute. I was sleeping around and doing things I never dreamed I would do. It was during this same year that I went on my search for spiritual truth.

Slone came to stay with me over the summer. He joined a youth group that summer. We both seemed to be treading lightly, careful not to slip into turmoil again. Not long after being there, he started asking if he could live with me again. I wanted to scream "YES!" but I did not want to do the wrong thing again—and I did not know what the right thing was.

I didn't know if I could trust myself. My drinking had me secretly worried. Not only was I drinking too often, but a strange new behavior had started. If I drank anything at all, I could not seem to stop. I would be at a party and find myself drinking anything and everything I could get my hands on. If it didn't have a cigarette butt floating in it, I was drinking it! My private loss of dignity seemed out of my control at that point. Each morning after, I would declare to myself that I'd only drink two drinks the next time, but the overdrinking would happen again.

Slone brought up the subject of living with me again one night, and in talking about it, he burst into tears. I could see him tearing in half as he said, "I don't know what to do! I want to live in both places at the same time!" The effect that my mistakes had on him was becoming more than I could watch. For several weeks I thought about what to do. I wanted him with me so badly, but if being a good mother meant recognizing that I was not a good mother and letting him live with his father, then that's what I had to do.

Then I sat him down one day in the living room, and I apologized for every poor choice I'd made with him. He would try to assure me that I didn't need to do this, but through tears I asked him to let me. When I was done, he hugged me and sincerely forgave me.

I vowed to myself to never let things get out of hand with him again. There was a newness in the air, and a cloud had lifted. He moved back to Nashville and was now headed for his teens. There were still many challenges to grow out of and overcome. I had not suddenly become June Cleaver, and he was no Wally, but I felt that we had just scaled an enormous mountain. I felt we were triumphant! I was so proud of us.

I lay there in my bed staring up at Rona, knowing that I was defeated before she ever walked into the room. The last thing on earth I wanted at a time like this was to spend one second away from Slone. I wanted him glued to my side. "The only game of Slone's that I've ever missed was while I was in surgery! And Slone is not out of control!" I shot back. "Oh!" she said. "I'm sorry. I just assumed that you were not able to take off work to go see his games."

She went on to plead her case, and I could read between the lines of it all. I could tell that Slone had been primed, and he was itching to do this. He would get the opportunity to play football and basketball with his cousin in Texas. This affirmed the ugly gut feeling I'd been having about being forced to go back to Texas. I threw in the towel and began to make plans in my mind for how and when. "Well, the truth is," I said, "I've been feeling like I'm going to have to move back to Texas anyway." She threw her head back and laughed a loud, victorious laugh.

I know my sister. She thrives on family interaction. Actually, Rona loves interaction with anything capable of conversation, but she has a special partiality to the sense of family. I know she was thrilled at the thought of having another family member within reach of her own nest.

From where I stood though, in that moment, sinking in a pool of utter dread, it played for me as if her laughter was coming out of the mouth of the Wicked Witch of the West. "Aaaaa hah hah hah haaah! I'll get you, my pretty!" She swooped in and snatched my baby boy up out of his bedroom, stuffed him in her basket, and pedaled off into the air on her little flying bike! Things could not have felt more out of control.

Nashville

What was it about Nashville? Why was I so drawn to and attached to this place? I'd asked myself that a thousand times, but the question was never more important than during this period. It certainly wasn't the music business. Months before my baptism, I'd come home one day after a frustrating meeting with my publisher. I walked in the door of the apartment, threw my guitars on the couch, and fell to my knees, saying, "I give up. This is obviously not what I am supposed to be doing with my life. If You will just show me, God, I will do it. I will burn these guitars and never sing another note if you will just show me what it is I am supposed to be doing down here!" I was so sick of it all. Music Row was one big back-stabbing high school cheerleading squad with the power to generate massive amounts of fame and money.

When I was about 7 years old, I took my mother's world atlas and drew a line from the northern panhandle of Texas, where I grew up, to Nashville, Tennessee. I skipped a couple of states getting there because each state was on a different page, but this was my magic carpet ride so, the exact route was irrelevant. To this day I don't totally understand why.

I didn't really like country music when I was a kid. It will forever hold a bad association for me, overshadowed by a date stamp of divorce and childhood turmoil.

My grandfather took me to see Tanya Tucker during her first year of touring. She never made it to the stage, though, due to a severe sore throat. They offered an autograph if you wanted to line up outside her bus. My grandfather insisted, and I couldn't disappoint the excitement in his eyes by telling him I wasn't really all that interested. The whole thing seemed like a worthless hassle to me. We stood in line, and there seemed to be some sort of uncomfortable tension mounting inside the bus. Finally the door opened, and a man stepped out. He explained that she simply did not feel well enough to even give autographs.

I hung my un-autographed picture of her on the wall at the foot of my bed. I remember staring at it and wondering what it must be like to be her. I had childhood asthma, and I couldn't imagine being dragged around like that and pushed to perform, sick or not. I felt very sorry for her.

The only thing of any influence for me that ever came out of Nashville was an eight-track tape of Jessi Colter. I was fixated on it. I would stare at the picture of her leaning back on that piano, with her long black hair flowing and wearing that big silver bracelet. While listening to her haunting vocal on songs like "Storms Never Last," I found a characteristic packed inside her voice like nothing I'd ever heard. There was something about her that seemed to perfectly define everything I wanted to be. Almost any other time I heard country music, it seemed to strike a bothersome chord within me.

My mother somehow got her hands on a pedal steel guitar at one point. It was solid silver, and I was in awe, watching her as she moved the slide and bent and plucked away at it in the living room for a short-lived stint. I was equally drawn to the emanating cry of pedal steel on the Colter eight-track. Mom never got much more than a few Hawaiian-sounding licks out of it. Rona and I would pretend to grass-skirt dance, and we would giggle as she played it. But secretly, I wanted her to get good at it so I could sing Jessi Colter songs to it. I don't know why she gave it up or where it went.

After the conversation with my sister about Slone, I sat staring out my bedroom window and asking myself that question again: *What is it about this place that keeps me in its grip?* I loved the landscape and terrain of Tennessee. There was something healing about it for me. I realized as I stared out into the evergreens that I had found a therapeutic hideaway in the trees and hills there. I had found God there. I couldn't stand the thought of leaving.

Faith

Mom and I went in to meet the oncologist and set the appointment for the next surgery. The plan was to open me up like the hood of a car and start yanking stuff out and sending it off. Although I was physically dreading this surgery with a passion, I was surprisingly at peace. A strange thing was happening to me. I felt as if I was in a constant state of spiritual awareness. I felt as if I had taken two steps up out of the material world and was walking on some invisible plane inside this protective bubble I had gotten caught up in during the experience of that first night.

After recovering a bit more, I had ventured out on my own to meet Cassie and Cynthia for dinner one night at one of my favorite Mexican restaurants. I had a moment where I looked at them, aware of this constant spiritual sensation. I felt that I was peering out at them from within the bubble. I actually wondered for a scary split second if maybe I had really died but "Saint Peter" just hadn't told me the whole truth yet. Maybe paradise plays out for a while as if nothing has happened.

I laughed at myself for stopping to contemplate such a thing, but this feeling of being on some other plane and looking at everything through the glass seemed unshakable. Even though this dwelling I'd found myself locked in was, no doubt, keeping me saturated in that "peace that passes understanding," I was still fighting to reclaim normal life.

I sat at the end of the examining table once again, staring at the floor in silence waiting for the oncologist to finally take the stage. Mom sat in a chair, arms crossed, rubbing her four fingers over her mouth the way she does when there is nothing she can do to fix a situation.

The doctor came in and introduced herself to my mother. Then she whirled around to look at me and stopped in her tracks. A look of confusion came over her face. She squinted her eyes at me and said, "Wow! You...you look incredible for someone who's been through what you've been through." She looked at the infamous manila folder for a moment and then said, "I'll tell you what. I'm not going to need to do an examination today. I want to just meet with you in the conference room briefly. My assistant will be in to show you the way in a moment." Then she walked out.

In the conference room I spotted a bookcase. While we were still waiting on the oncologist to join us, I got up and walked over to it. I grabbed the book with the most appropriate title and started digging through the index. Mom and I had done quite a bit of research by that time. We'd looked into every possible cure out there, from a well-balanced diet to coffee enemas. She had even sat with me, her face melting into dreadful, empathetic furrows as she watched me try to choke down shots of wheat grass. I was curious to see what the medical journals housed in an actual oncologist's office might say about my "mild case of cancer."

The oncologist walked in and caught me. I nonchalantly returned the book to the shelf before finding the cure. She pulled a chair up beside her for me to sit in and opened up the mysterious file folder. The folder tab read, "Jill Riley, Ovarian Cancer." She began pointing things out within the details of the pages. "You have so many things going on at once. You have this scar tissue from prior surgeries, and you have this scar tissue from endometriosis, and one of the tumors that we found actually ..." Her voice trailed off, and most of what she was saying was not fully registering, because I was still engrossed in the tab title. I did take note of how she marveled over my sad set of circumstances as if I were an impossible algebraic formula she was destined to crack. She caught me staring at the tab. "It is officially termed ovarian cancer, but don't let that throw you," she said.

"What I've decided to do is postpone this surgery. I think I want to monitor this with CAT scans for a while before proceeding with the next surgery." I couldn't believe my ears! After everything she'd just gone over, that was the last thing I thought I'd hear. *No way!* I thought. I felt as if I had just received word straight from heaven that my prayers had been answered and I had been released!

I had been reading the book of James. It was a random book I picked to read out of my new Bible. At least, I thought at the time that it was random. It instructed anyone who was sick to go to the elders and be anointed with oil. I wasn't sure who "the elders" were, but I was pretty sure it was the old people in the church. I called the church and asked if I could meet with an elder. I explained my situation, and I was invited to come up on a Monday night and stand in line outside the door of a classroom. Three of the sweetest elderly men eventually welcomed me in. They stood over me, put oil on my head, and fervently prayed to God for healing. I loved that they did this behind closed doors. There was nothing showy about it. It was just pure and simple faith on the part of these men.

I walked out of the oncologist's office feeling as if I could fly. I began telling people that we were not monitoring cancer. We were monitoring faith. The truth was that at times I had fear the size of a mountain and faith the size of a mustard seed, but I knew God was enlarging that faith in me. He was giving me the faith of those elders, and this was just the beginning. I really didn't understand all of this olive oil business, but I knew the God of the Bible was in this with me, and He could be trusted. I was just trying to be obedient. That is faith.

Kicking against the Goads

I made the decision to move back to Texas. Slone was already there, and I was surrendered to that decision. Mom had gone back to Texas, and I stayed alone in Nashville for a few weeks to tie up loose ends and pack up the apartment. As far as I could tell, this was a permanent move. Maybe I was done with Nashville, and maybe Nashville was done with me. I had finally started getting good at writing songs. I was a terribly inconsistent artist, because of the lack of time I was able to put into it as a working single mother. My band and I had been playing a semi-regular gig downtown, though, and it was finally beginning to gel.

There was a new stirring around my music just before I was diagnosed that had even placed me in the coveted position of having several producers and production companies pursuing me at once. There is obvious negotiating power in that position. As burnt out on near record deals as I had become, I was getting excited again because these were not Music Row producers.

These were the inspired, creative people that can be found in the fringe there. They have nothing against fame or fortune or those who go after it. They are just more driven by creativity itself. They genuinely believed in what they were hearing and wanted to offer a springboard. This was what I had been waiting so long for. Once these producers got word that I was leaving town, one by one, gently and quietly, they all moved on. I couldn't blame any of them. As I met with each one, they were all genuinely supportive. My situation was just too unstable to build on at that point.

I sat in my apartment, dreading the move. Combing through the memories of my time in Nashville, I realized the problem. It wasn't music, even though music was in me and would not leave me alone. It wasn't the trees and rivers and lakes, even though to this day I can think of them and still pine a little. It was that I had accidentally become family with the girls of The Gang.

Cynthia and Cassie had been by my side whether in person, over the phone, or in spirit, every single step of the way through this. Alicia, JK, Randi, Vaughan, Rebecca, Beth, Michele, and so many others continued to go out of their way to surround me with support. It was unthinkably hard to walk away from that. I didn't really know the power of that until I felt forced to let go of it.

Over the years, these girls had supplied a kind of connection that I needed. They knew me for who I had become and left room for who I was becoming. I had grown more as a person through the relationships I had with these women than through any other thing.

They provided a place for me to push the boundaries of my deep-rooted trust issues. They confronted me and pressed until things got worked out. They talked behind my back, regularly, in an effort to find the best way to tell me when I was in need of change. They knew how to hurt my feelings without harming me. They instinctively handled my woundedness with authentic grace and understanding.

These girls were artists, and artists seem to have a unique understanding of the wounded.

Cynthia's cultivating and encouraging nature was something like a scalpel splitting open my locked-up emotions. Cassie stood beside her, hovering over me with her surgeon's light shining from her forehead. She was reaching in, digging for my hidden spirit, pulling parts of it out, and saying, "Aha! See, here it is!"

These friendships didn't come without tough love when it was needed. Randi called me one day, and even though she and I weren't all that close, she was the one who had the guts to say, "OK, Jill, enough is enough! Why are you still smoking after being diagnosed with cancer?" Randi was a headstrong Jewish-mother type who grew up in New York. You always knew where you stood with her. When Randi said this, it was as if the hammer of a bell whacked the inside of my skull. It was humiliating and embarrassing, and it offended the life out of me.

I went home that day and got so angry—not at Randi, but at the fact that I could not quit smoking. Debbie Eaton, my drummer's wife, had once said, "Jill, your lungs are your wings!" These two statements rang in my head until I wanted to scream. I hated the fact that something had such control over me.

I had so much anger in me that I felt I could put my fist through the wall if I punched it. I shouted, "God! I have tried and tried to quit smoking, and You know it! I cannot do it, and if You want me to quit, You are going to have to do it Yourself!" I wasn't sure how, or even if God responded to that kind of irreverent and disrespectful behavior, but I didn't care.

Two days later, a woman I had never met sent me two books by way of her daughter. Her daughter was a new friend of mine. I didn't get to see her that often but she was a dear friend. The first book was called *The Journey*. The other was *Alan Carr's Easy Way to Quit Smoking*. I read the latter over the following weekend, and other than one time, four months later, I have not smoked since. Apparently God answers even irreverent prayers.

As much as I was struggling with moving away from the girls, I think I also knew deep down that I was in need of an official departure from The Gang. We had all shared our complacency and ambiguous thoughts about God, and I had personally reveled in the freedom of it. But my so-called freedom had taxed me. I felt a beckoning, whether I liked it or not, so I continued to surrender to it. In the end I decided to leave my furniture in storage in Nashville. It just seemed like too much of a commitment too soon to move it all to Texas.

My dad offered me a room at his house. There was no room at Rona's, where Slone was staying, but everyone lives a few miles from each other, and we would just have to make it work. I called my dad and told him of my decision to store my stuff in Nashville. With a supportive smile in his tone, he told me he wasn't surprised and had been half waiting for the call.

A couple of weeks before leaving Nashville, one of the girls was having a party, and I decided to go. I was worn out, but it would be one of my last chances to hang out with them. I had been there a while and was about to walk out the door, when a guy that I'd met when I first moved to Nashville walked up and looked right at me. "Wow! The last time I saw you," he said, "you were blowing me away at the Bluebird Café." I felt immediately embarrassed for the guy, because he obviously had the wrong guitar-toting brunette. I didn't respond, giving him a second to catch his mistake.

"Yeah, Jill Riley! I don't know if we've ever met before. I'm Jim Kimball." I was confused. "Yeah, I called your publisher and tried to set up an appointment. I wanted to produce you, but I could never get that to come together." He obviously hadn't mistaken me for someone else, but I didn't know what he was talking about. Now I was blown away. How was it that I had a producer pursuing me at some point and I was never made aware of it?

He started probing for musical vital signs, so I quickly let him off the hook by explaining that I was moving back to Texas in a few days. Out of politeness, it seemed, he half-heartedly talked about the possibility of "internet writing." Writing via email was becoming a fairly normal practice.

Then, to my surprise, without any apparent flirtation in his tone, he invited me to breakfast the next morning to discuss the possibility of writing and to fill me in on the story about contacting my publisher. I could see the wheels turning in his little producer head. There's a look they get. Not that it mattered by then, but my curiosity about what had happened between him and my publisher was killing me. God forbid I leave town missing yet another thing to be bitter and disappointed about in Music Row! My ego still had its cravings, and I didn't see any harm in a little boost. It would be my parting gift to myself.

The Master Builder

$\mathcal{S}$omething of destiny seemed to settle on us as we walked around Radnor Lake after breakfast. I think it started the moment chill bumps rose as he recited the lyrics to a song of his called "Song for Clara." There was a mystical feeling that was permeating even over and above the bubble experience. We both knew something was stirring. You know musical chemistry when you see it, and it was blinding that day. I could hardly think about it, because I was too tired of clinging to sugar cubes under water. There had never been a time when I was so dead inside to the idea of doing anything noteworthy with my music. My future was such an unsure blur that I didn't have it in me to even begin to think in these terms. But I was connecting with his creativity. I couldn't help myself. Before the end of the day, he was my new producer and walking through a sudden rainstorm, we both rolled up our sleeves to take in the lethal injection of boy producer meets girl singer/songwriter romance.

It would be harder than ever to leave now, but I loaded my bags into the car and took off for Dallas. I threw my chin in the air and decided to "keep on keepin' on" by booking local coffee house gigs. I was starting to feel a little steam inside from the idea of stirring up a local following and working on a new record with Jim. I had decided to stick with the team of doctors I had in Nashville rather than transferring everything to Texas. It would be necessary for me to go back to Nashville occasionally for the CAT scans. Jim and I had a plan to record during those visits.

I played my first coffee house in downtown Fort Worth. My sister and mother came out to support me. Rona rallied some friends to come out. There was a terrible lonesome and hollow cry in my sound. It happens on occasion, and it's too painful for people to sit through. I didn't have the energy to switch the channel inside myself and perform. As I sang I realized that playing coffee houses in Texas was not going to fill this enormous void inside of me. I wasn't sure anything ever would. I packed up the equipment and cried my way back to my dad's. I didn't stop crying. If I was in Texas, I was crying. I was lost. I was never lonelier. I was dying.

On one of my first visits back to Nashville I went to meet the girls for dinner. Calina, a fairly new "inductee," introduced herself. I had known of her, but we hadn't ever spent time together. She knew of my story, and she gave me a book called *Love, Medicine and Miracles*.

I didn't even know this girl, and she'd written a personal, encouraging note inside the front cover. She also invited me to a Bible study. I knew the minute she asked me that God was telling me to go. The Bible study was hosted by Van Stephenson and his wife, Karen. Van was a songwriter and member of the band Blackhawk. I had met him a few years before. I distinctly remembered him as a humble, subdued type. I had no idea he was a Christian. Van had been battling cancer for a while when he and his wife decided to host this weekly gathering. I attended that week before I went back to Texas. I told them I would join them anytime I was in town.

My first CAT scan was reported to be perfect. I was back in Texas when my oncologist called me personally. She explained that she didn't normally do that, but she was so happy for me that she decided to call herself. I had mixed emotions. I was elated that nothing was found, but at the same time, if it was perfect, what was I doing back in Texas? I continued to keep myself in limbo, scrounging for odd jobs and low-paying gigs. So many people had helped me out financially, and I hated being this kind of burden.

Committing to any full-time job was too much for me. I just could not dig my heels that far into the dirt of Texas yet. I was on the phone with someone from Nashville around the clock. If I wasn't on the phone or computer with someone from Nashville, it only meant I was on the road back there. With the news of the perfect CAT scan, I needed to make a decision about what I was doing next and then move on. My family was getting fed up and feeling taken advantage of. I could feel it. I was trapped.

A couple of months passed. I woke up one morning with fairly severe abdominal pain. It never let up, so I called my oncologist's office that afternoon and described what was going on. She urged me to fly up to Nashville right away. They ran a sonogram, and very clearly I could see the outline of a sizable mass with two smaller masses attached. The technician was zooming in on and measuring these places.

My oncologist went over the scans with me and explained there was an orange-sized mass on the colon. It was potentially penetrating the colon and causing the problem. She explained she would need to operate as soon as possible. She would be calling on the help of a colon specialist to assist her in surgery and would need me to meet with him. She also broke the news that this surgery would more than likely result in a permanent colostomy. If not permanent, it would require at least a six-month colostomy.

I sat at the end of the examination table, numb and checked out, watching her lips move up and down. I left her office and calmly drove directly to the nearest restaurant that served my brand of tequila. I ordered two shots and called Cynthia. I told her the news, and she assured me she would get the girls together and have them there in no time. Then I called Jim.

I don't remember calling my mom. I guess I did. I'm not sure. I remember getting a call from her after several shots. I don't remember what was said. I remember wearing Cassie's taco hat and staring out from under it at Jim, who'd joined the strange party as well. I was wondering what in the world I had gotten this poor man into. I remember everyone being so tolerant of my unacceptable behavior. If just for a moment I could stop and get off this riddled life of mine. At times I would wake up in the morning, and seconds would go by before I would remember the "cancer." In those seconds I didn't have "cancer," and I hated it when those seconds were gone.

After hearing the news, Beth Hooker wanted to pass this comforting bit of wisdom on to me. She told not to sweat it. "The worst thing about having a colostomy bag," she said, "is finding shoes to match!" I thought that was hilarious in contrast to all the doom, and I couldn't wait to use this line!

I watched the colon specialist as he scratched out a cocktail-napkin style drawing of his plan on a note pad. He again warned me of the likely permanent colostomy, and then, without the slightest bit of hesitation, he showed me that part of the plan was to cut out, along with a large portion of my colon, the top half of the vagina! At a complete loss for any and every thing to say in response to such a horrific proposal, I whipped out the "shoes to match" line. This man looked at me as if I had gone mad right there before his eyes.

Maybe I had. I couldn't comprehend what he'd just said, and there was no way I could actually tell anybody about this. How humiliated did I have to be before all of this was going to end?

Something even more frightening was looming, though, and I was just about to come out of my skin all together. I had not been able to shake a constant nagging feeling that I was not supposed to have *any* surgery. I don't recall exactly when it started, but I know it was almost immediately after we looked at the sonogram. This feeling was getting stronger and stronger. I kept checking myself, because there was no doubt that I didn't want to have this surgery. I would question myself on whether it was some form of denial or running away.

Somehow, I knew this feeling was separate from all of those feelings, though. Yes, I did want to run, and I could even rationalize and defend reasons for at least postponing the surgery. I'd had cysts in the past that came and went. So, who was to say this wasn't just another cyst?

The day after drowning myself in tequila, I called my mom to apologize and assure her it was a one-time reaction. I had just come to my wit's end in all of it, but I would be OK. I told her in that conversation that we weren't sure that it wasn't just a cluster of cysts. I purposely played it down, because I needed to soften it and prime her in case I decided not to have the surgery. I had actually asked the oncologist what she thought the chances were of it simply being cysts. She gave me one of those "You let me handle this" looks and said there was no way to know. But, she explained, in light of my recent history, and due to the "cloudiness" and the speed of the growth of these masses, she was unwavering in her decision to remove them.

When a child is sick, the mother wants it fixed right then and there! I understood this, and on one hand, I felt the same way. I wanted this thing gone, even if that meant surgery, no matter how much I dreaded it! But this notion was pressing, and I finally couldn't hold it in anymore.

I got the guts up to tell Cynthia. Her eyes widened, and she said, "Oh my gosh, Jill! Vaughan and I have been talking, and we are feeling the same thing!" Her words came like a burst of affirmation, and I knew right then that I was not going to have this surgery. It was everything to have them, not only supportive of it, but also in agreement with it in their spirits. That is a powerful thing, and I have since come to know that God works through this power of agreement in amazing ways.

The girls rallied like never before. I was staying with Cynthia. At the time Cynthia was renting from her friend Sharon, who had houses in L.A., Nashville, and New York. Sharon was only in Nashville a few times a year. They could not have been more hospitable to me. Sharon offered her empty room any time I needed it.

After hours of pacing Sharon's Mexican tile, I finally mustered up the guts to call the colon specialist. I didn't have a clue how to explain this inner knowing I was convinced of, so I just told him I was getting a second opinion, because actually I *was* getting a "second opinion." I told him I would call him back and let him know when I had made my final decision. He said, frankly, "Jill, I know what you are doing. You are trying to wish this away, and this is not something that can be postponed." I told him I understood and appreciated his concern, but I had to do this. I couldn't put myself through the conversation with the oncologist, so I asked him to pass the information along to her.

Cynthia was out of town for a few days, so I had the house to myself. I sat in a chair in Sharon's peaceful living room, staring out at the trees once again. The sun was going down, so the greens were changing shades. I said to God,

"OK, I've done it!" I knew all along that it was God pushing me to do this. I hadn't heard any thundering voice or seen any writing on the wall, but there was no doubt where it was coming from. I did not want to be a person who ran around telling people how they had been "heeeealed in the name of Jeee-sus!!" It just wasn't me. God knew this. We'd made several deals before I committed to coming into His camp. I wasn't going to be that kind of Christian.

I wasn't ashamed of Christianity anymore, and I would boldly tell anyone that I had concluded that it was the religion of the one true God, but we had an agreement that I absolutely would not ever become a radical type. People like me run screaming from Christianity due to the radicals. I was never convinced that God had a handle on how to effectively reach His people down here. It seemed to me that He was a little out of touch. I was dead serious about this arrogant opinion of mine, but at this point, I felt as if God had me by the collar.

I was not happy with or in God at that point. I was in a fight with Him, and I was not winning. He seemed relentless to me, but I wasn't about to cross Him. I had always hated the phrase "the fear of God," but I now had it. He seemed to have control, and I had no say in it. I also knew deep down what this was really all about, and I couldn't believe He was actually going to do this to me. I had been fighting him all summer long in Texas because I knew what He was up to, but He was not taking no for an answer. The latest sonogram was proof of that. He meant business with me!

Strangely, I also still had this trust in Him that I'd never had in anyone or anything. The trust was as unshakable as the fear. I sipped my coffee in quiet surrender for a long time. Then I said, "OK, I've walked away from the doctors, but I can't just sit here and do nothing! You have to give me something to do." I was tired, and when I was in Nashville I slept like a baby. I went upstairs and passed out.

The next morning, even before I was completely awake, I heard "Read! Read! Read!" very clearly in my mind. I stopped mid stretch, because it struck me that those words were connected to no other thought of mine. Those words were not connected to me at all. That was a specific verbal instruction coming from outside of myself. It was God telling me what I was supposed to do. He was verbally answering my request from the night before.

That very day, it seemed, people began handing me books right and left. It was almost as if a stack of books fell from the sky and landed at my feet as I sat in that same chair reading them. Following my gut instincts, the first book I opened was the other book that my friend had passed on to me called *The Journey* by Brandon Bays.

My Journey

This book was astonishing, and the timing of my reading it was perfect. Like me, the author of this book had felt led to walk away from any suggested surgery to remove an abdominal tumor. In her case, though, the tumor was actually the size of a basketball. God knew I needed to be one-upped in faith, and this woman certainly did that. She did not profess to be a Christian. The book was endorsed by Deepak Chopra and used the language of New Age and the healing arts. Even though I had abandoned this type of reading, I was convinced that this was the leading of the same God of the Bible that I had been following to this point.

This book affirmed that God was up to what I feared most. I had a closet full of secrets and skeletons. The door had been bulging for years, and any time I walked by it, I'd kick it shut again. Any time I had to be in Texas, I was too close to that closet. This book actually suggested that a tumor can sometimes be connected to deep emotional wounds and the inability to forgive. This seemed absurd at first, and I didn't buy into it at all. It seemed like New Age mumbo-jumbo, but I knew that this book was God's way of telling me that it was time to face the closet.

Once when I was a senior in high school, I was sitting at a red light on an ordinary afternoon when I suddenly had a flashback. I was shocked at what I saw, and my instant response was, "I don't know where that memory has been, but it's going back there!" I shut it out of my mind, and the memory never returned until four years later. I was 22 when Rona had asked me an innocent question about something that had happened in our childhood. The door to that closet opened wide and started spilling out, as flashes of several instances of childhood sexual abuse ran through my head. I could not shut the door again to save my life.

Rona didn't realize what she had sparked. I fought it hard for a few months. It was at that point that I began kicking the closet door shut. My motto became: "That ruined my childhood, and I'll be damned if I let it ruin my adulthood!"

The night before we discovered the orange-sized mass, a strange thing happened that I was beginning to understand as I read this book. I had another flashback out of nowhere, but this one was bizarre. I didn't understand the reason for it, but it was so vivid that I couldn't ignore it. I was sitting on Jim's couch, and I just let it play out on the screen of my mind. Jim was working in the studio. In the flashback, I was about 9 years old, and I had little French braids in my hair. I was supposed to be getting ready to take a bath, so I was flopping around the bathroom in my underwear like Gilda Radnor's little girl character from *Saturday Night Live*. I looked in the bath and saw a bug. I called for mom and asked her if she could come get the bug out. She looked at the bug and said, "Oh! That's a silverfish. He'll eat your clothes if we don't get him!" I remembered thinking in my little-girl mind that this tiny bug could eat my entire closet full of clothes. That was the end of the memory.

I sat there on the couch thinking, *That was weird!* I went into Jim's bedroom to lie down for a minute. A book on his nightstand caught my attention. I'd never noticed it before. It was by Louise Hay. I'd read a little of her stuff in the days of my searching. The book was called *Heal Your Body*, and as I read one page out of it, a power swept over me. I was hoping Jim would not walk in and catch me in my condition—it was overwhelming, and reading it was actually making me quiver. Tears were rolling, and I was stunned by what the page knew about me. I don't remember now exactly what I read. I just remember that it was hitting some nail on the head.

I came to understand that the "bug in the bath" memory caused me to see, for the first time in over 20 years, that I had actually once been an innocent, pure, and beautiful little girl. I had not known that little girl. I only knew the hardened, desperate, tough girl who chain-smoked, cussed, drank, and stood guard. She was completely unattractive in contrast to the beauty of that 9 year old. It was as if the tough girl had shoved this little girl into that same closet and said, "You shut up and let me handle this!" It was a daunting revelation.

It was important that I discover this little girl. She was the person God had created, not this mangled, thrashed thing I'd become. That is what the world around me had created. Even the Bible said, "Unless you change, and become like little children, you will never enter into the kingdom of heaven" (Matthew 18:3 NIV). I had to get back to the little girl, and I had to get the little girl back to God! Jim Kimball was a child in a grown man's body, and he was placed in my life, if for no other reason, than to teach me how to be free in adult-sized shoes. He walked in a state of wonder and amazement and appreciation. He was full of life. I was full of death. God had set me up. The more I read Brandon Bays' story, sitting alone in that chair, the more I knew God had my back, and I loved Him more deeply than ever.

As much as I didn't want to be dragged back through the stuff of childhood, I knew God was assuring me that He would not lead me to dig in details that were either too painful or were simply irrelevant. It became evident that He was only bringing to my mind memories of things that ultimately set a destructive pattern in my life, memories of things that caused me to hate. So I allowed Him. I went on long walks and drives. I sat in the chair. I read and read and read.

Cassie sat with me one night and listened to my entire story from start to finish. This may have been the most healing step of the whole journey for me. I had never told anyone the whole story. When I was done, we looked at each other and laughed. "Dang! No wonder I'm so screwed up!" I said. I was overwhelmed by the effect of the A to Z version of my story.

You don't really know what you've been through until you inventory your life like that. I felt an undeniable shifting in the area of the mass. I will never forget it. The next day I split an apricot in half to eat it. The seed inside it was shriveled to one quarter its original size. It felt as if it was a little sign. I didn't share that with anyone, because I also felt it sounded a little crazy!

Cynthia came back to town and joined right in the process. Cynthia is one of the greatest listeners I've ever met, but at the same time you didn't really need to explain yourself to her. She is in tune and has a way of knowing you better than you knew yourself sometimes. When any one of the girls was down, she was always the first to come to the rescue. We talked for hours about how I should proceed.

We had dubbed Alicia our token "stage mother" simply because she wasn't a musician or songwriter. She was another nurturing type, and I loved to be with her. If you were with Alicia you were having fun, and that was all there was to it. However, Alicia had suddenly hit a bump in the road, and we just couldn't stand for it. Our good friend had broken up with her. Cynthia and I took it upon ourselves to call him up and invite him to lunch. He agreed and we set the time. We would fix it all in no time.

When we showed up to lunch, he was with a new girl he was dating, so it was going to be a little bit difficult to properly straighten him out. I had second thoughts about whether I was in any state to be getting in the middle of this kind of codependent diversion in the first place, but something said "go."

In the middle of a polite and chatty conversation, the subject of my health came up. The new girlfriend immediately perked up. My sensors went on overload, and I could feel in the air that something was about to go down. She asked, "Which one of you is sick?" We gave a few more details of my condition, and to me she looked as if she wanted to come over the table but she was maintaining great restraint. "You really, really need to meet my roommate. She's a psychic healer. She can help you! You *really* need to come!" she urged.

Cynthia seemed willing to be supportive of whatever might work. As we all discussed it, I told them I would think about it, but I wasn't really planning to give it a second thought. As we left the restaurant, seemingly out of nowhere, I remembered that the last time I was there, I was introduced to a friend of a friend. We were all waiting on a table. To kill time, this girl began to show us muscle testing. I'd never seen it before.

She put a vitamin in my left hand, told me to press the middle finger of my right hand down on the index finger of my right hand, and feel the amount of tension. Then she replaced the vitamin in my left hand with a cigarette. She told me to repeat the pressing down and feel the difference. I couldn't believe how much weaker my right hand was. She explained that the body knows what it needs and what it doesn't need. It was a strange little experiment and even stranger that I suddenly remembered it as we were leaving. I guess God was forewarning me that I would soon run into this "muscle test girl" and to pay attention when I did.

Down the Rabbit Hole

*A*t this point on my path I began to feel as if I was walking through a car wash. Stuff was slapping me and shoving me around, but I couldn't fight all that off because water was blasting me in the face, and it took everything in me just to stay upright.

After Cynthia and I left the restaurant, without pressuring me, Cynthia explained that she felt a sense of urgency about me meeting with the psychic healer. She knew all about my experiences with the Ouija board and knew that I was steering clear of anything like that. But Cynthia seemed to be advising me out of a heart-felt desperation to get this taken care of for me.

Aside from what Cynthia thought; my ability to discern God's leading was becoming supernaturally sharp, and as crazy as it seemed, I was convinced He was giving me the go-ahead to do this. At first, I thought it was more like a test— one of those "Go ahead! Knock yourself out! See what you get?" sort of things. I wasn't about to fall for that. I was completely surrendered, falling in love with and becoming loyal to the God of the Bible. Though I couldn't have quoted the scriptures at the time, I knew that the Bible made it inarguably clear to never seek the counsel of a psychic or medium.

I told Cynthia I would think about it but that I did not have a good feeling about it. I continued to pray and continued to get this "green light" feeling from God. Even though this didn't line up with anything I knew about Christianity, and I didn't know one Christian who would be in agreement with the decision to do this, I was convinced that it was an instruction from God. Then I ran across a passage in the Bible that made it seem so simple: "Do not put out the Spirit's fire; do not treat prophecies with contempt. Test everything. Hold on to the good. Avoid every kind of evil" (1 Thessalonians 5:19-22 NIV).

I became convinced that God was leading me into this with a two-fold purpose. In her book, Brandon Bays described an exercise using a visual technique to bring about forgiveness. When I read it, I knew that God was going to make me do it. It was one of those things I would have made fun of in the past. As much as I wanted to be a hippie, I'd never gotten free enough from my cow-town roots to sit cross-legged, staring into the face of some long-haired Jim Morrison type, moving to the beat of bongos. The bottom line was that I was a simple country girl from the panhandle of Texas, and when it came down to it, I just wasn't made of that stuff. I needed tangibility to make me believe in a thing.

I had voluntarily walked into this war zone though, and the only hope I felt I had left was to stay wired to command central and follow His orders. While I was treading carefully through the land mines, I was determined, once and for all, to rid myself of a 20-year tormenting burden. This burden seemed to be the real root of all my trouble - no matter how deep I tried to bury it. This root was the fact that I hated my mother. My hate for her had been boiling and rising for years. At about the time the screaming whistle inside me was ready to blow, my brother was killed in a car accident, and I was thrown into the deepest empathy for her. I swallowed my overgrown hatred whole, and now, according to what God seemed to be showing me, it was killing me.

My mother was riddled with grief and guilt for as long as I could remember. It had felt impossible to step up to that grief and guilt and come to my own defense. Any thing that justified my mother though, could never lessen my own private pain, and Brandon Bays' book was telling me what God had been trying to get me to see for months. It was time to forgive. In order to forgive I would have to revisit some things.

Time and time again I would think that I had forgiven her and let go of everything from my past, but that hatred would rise again. I remember once asking God in anger, "How many times do I have to forgive this!" Every experience of pain from my childhood seemed to hang inside of me on a hook of hatred for her.

The painful experiences were like articles of clothing hanging from that hook and the hook was about to give way under the weight of it all. This hook of hatred stemmed from one conversation with her when I was 14 years old. The conversation probably lasted less than fifteen minutes. That one small moment in time birthed this hook that I began hanging every cloak of burden on. It was time to finally face that conversation and do whatever it was that a person had to do to let go and forgive.

When I was 14, my mother sat me down in the living room to have a rare and awkwardly tense mother-daughter talk. The conversation subtly revealed that she had known of my struggles with sexual abuse. It dawned on me as she spoke that I had been carrying that secret in order to protect her, when ironically she, my own mother, had known and done nothing to protect me. What a fool I had been. As if that wasn't enough, her tone was clearly shaming and blaming me. My head was the only one the hammer was coming down upon in this ordeal. That hatred rose up in me that day and had been festering ever since. I was so infuriated I had nothing to say. In my mind, from then on, it was every bit her fault.

I started drinking alcohol when I was 13 because it was the sneaky thing to do. I had graduated to Crown Royal straight out of the bottle, which I kept hidden under the seat of my car. In our small farming community, not only were we allowed to drive underage, but most of us also had our own car by the time we were in seventh or eighth grade. I had an empty bottle collection in a certain ditch that shocks me now when I look back on it. I had walked away from the conversation about the sexual abuse only slightly more numb than normal. Life was a deadened blur. My first year of high school would prove to be the worst year of my life.

Not long after that conversation, I went "riding around," as we called it, by myself in my ugly lemon-yellow Comet. Everyone was out of town at a basketball game. My boyfriend was on the varsity team, and I thought I'd kill some time waiting for the basketball bus to pull into town. I took a swig from my secret bottle and noticed another car dragging Main Street. He was a friend from school, and he waved me over to talk near the school. I stopped and rolled my window down. He asked if I wanted to get in with him, and we'd ride around together while I was waiting.

There were a thousand people in that town. When someone dies, everyone grieves as if they've lost their own, because they have. The whole town was one big family. We never locked doors, not even when we left town. We slept on trampolines every night during the summer. We didn't necessarily have babysitters. Young kids often stayed alone at home all night. Everyone knew everything about everyone, or so they thought.

Boys did weird things. They always had. That was just the way it was. So much of it went ignored or accepted as simple pubescent conduct. Although this boy had a particularly unique habit, I remained naively unalarmed by it, because no one ever seemed concerned about boys and their strange behavior. Coaches openly made crude sexual comments. Men had blatantly encouraged their sons in the whole "coming of age" goings-on. Once, in a manipulative effort to have his way, a guy I had no relationship with tried to belittle me into his will by telling me I was just too young to understand that sex was what I was made for.

So, apart from the "Peeping-Tom" habit of this particular boy, which I assumed I should just ignore, this boy was something like an older brother to me. He was a talented, well-respected, and otherwise great kid. I didn't give his invitation a second thought. He asked if I had anything to drink. I held up the Crown bottle and then jumped in the car with him. I do not remember the gradual build of drunkenness. I had only had one swig from the bottle before I met up with him and wasn't even slightly buzzed when I got in his car. I only remember being in his car for a very short period of time and driving back toward Main Street. I remember something about the lid of the Crown Royal bottle.

The next thing I remembered was waking up, with no pants on, in the backseat of his car and realizing what was about to happen. I was too weak to move my arms or legs. It was like screaming in a dream. I could only muster a whispering shout, "No!" I was crying inside and begging him with my eyes, but I could see a look in his eyes warning me that if I fought, he would fight back—and I would lose. I became acutely aware of the choice I had, and I willfully chose defeat. I would deal with a plaguing guilt from that decision for years to come. I felt as if I was drowning inside myself. Clearly I had been drugged, but even if I hadn't been, I'm not sure I had the fight in me anymore. I was still a virgin, but just about everything except intercourse had already been imposed on me.

The drugs had taken a strange effect, and things seemed a bit psychedelic. I remember bits and pieces of my own strange behavior. The mind game was staggering. As the rape continued, rather than suffocating in the anguish of it, I turned a corner in my mind and decided to accept that this was just who I was. In and out of lucidity, I lost myself in this first-time sexual experience and took it on as if I could somehow conquer it by accommodating the degradation. I would be a victor one way or the other, even in the midst of all the defeat. I accepted the disgrace, and in twisted indignation, I wore it like a crown. I don't remember it ending, or my leaving there or getting home. I shoved the memory into that closet and shut the door.

It was time to open the bulging door and finally face it all, head-on. No matter what I thought of God's approach, he had me cornered, and I couldn't find a way out except to turn around and have that devastating surgery. I couldn't get over the cruel irony of the surgery. In doing some research, I had read that some medical scientists believe that in some cases endometriosis is caused from sexual activity before the female body is fully developed, causing a retardation of the female organs. The lining of the uterus begins to disperse in the wrong direction, causing scar tissue to build up. Over time, the abdominal cavity is a complete, painful mess.

In turning back to Christ I had become convicted about my casual sex life and I had been trying, unsuccessfully, to refrain from sex. A sex life, according to my previous standards, had become something to be maintained. It was not much different from an exercise routine. It was an item on the task list that regularly needed to be taken care of.

It was never hard to find a willing partner in the music business. Creating music is an intimate thing. Songwriters walk around inside out, and this element of Nashville causes a kind of coed locker-room feel within the creative community. This element is hard on introverted loners— and marriages.

Aside from any crutch I could lean on from the past, I had willingly taken on this lifestyle all on my own in Nashville. I had lowered myself beyond reach, and my heart was beginning to yell for help from the bottom of that pit. I was appalled by the fact that I had now knowingly treated sex with no more respect and sensitivity than my childhood perpetrators. I hated that I could never have sex with one man without knowing of the list of all the others. Nothing was sacred about the act of sex, and I had always so desperately needed it to be.

I couldn't understand this need at the time. Why was it that I needed sex to be something sacred? What does it even mean to be sacred? Why is it that whenever one sexual partner cheats on another it deeply hurts the other, no matter what moral standards are involved? What were these unspoken laws all about? It wasn't just me. Every movie seemed to be about this. Every country song sings this same theme over and over again. Why don't we listen? Why can't we see this? The whole world preaches this sermon every minute of every hour of every day!

The summer after that harrowing first year of high school, we moved to my grandfather's ranch about an hour from where we had been living. I spent that summer alone, learning to play guitar in the endless canyons that surrounded our house. My confidant and sounding board was a beautiful, steadfast, and protective Quarter Horse. He carried my burdens and let me fly free upon his back.

Soon after school started, I fell in love for the first time with a boy named Kirk Welch. He was equally infatuated. We eventually progressed to being sexually active, and while it was clearly wrong, it would remain a benchmark in my mind of being the closest thing to sacred sex I would ever get to experience in my life.

His father had died when he was 11, and he had been nurtured through the grief by his mother and sister, two of the warmest and most caring women I'd ever been around. His stepfather was a fun-loving yet firm, upright, and respectable man. I believe this combination created a temperament in him that proved to be the perfect healing recipe for me.

His family took me in as if I was one of them. My world was in the palm of his hand, and though I never fully realized it then, I was so thankful for him and his family. Kirk was my true friend and I was his. I never told him the secret details of the past, and he had no way of knowing what a refuge I was finding in our friendship and the warmth and acceptance of his loving family. People often ask, "Where was God?" When I began to look back on it, I could see so clearly that God was right there surrounding me in the aftermath with all of this - the canyons, the music, the quarter horse and these wonderful relationships.

Though I was able to run into the restoring arms of these things for a season, I still continued to feed on the poison of hate and anger. Over time, this poison had done its work and sonograms and CAT scans were revealing that I had become as much a physical wreck as I was an emotional wreck. It was beginning to make sense to me that the two could possibly be connected. I had done all I knew to do in order to forgive the past. I didn't seem to know the magic combination. This forgiveness exercise the book described seemed critical.

There was one coincidental clue at lunch that day with the psychic healer's roommate. She described a very similar forgiveness exercise and explained it was part of the session. I finally became convinced that God was telling me that I was fully capable of cutting through any New Age nonsense and getting whatever I needed out of a session with this so-called healer. Apparently, it was this silly little forgiveness exercise. So, I finally agreed to meet with her.

Planet Earth

*A*t our initial appointment, the psychic healer and I discussed what she planned to do so I could decide whether or not I wanted to proceed. Cynthia offered to go to the appointment with me, maybe as much out of her own curiosity as support for me. When we entered the psychic's apartment we introduced ourselves, and we were offered tea and shown to the couch. There was nothing eerie or spooky about it. I felt very relaxed, and the conversation stayed light and ordinary. But soon after I sat down on the couch, the psychic healer looked behind and above me. Her head pulled away slightly in surprise, and her eyes widened in what looked to be authentic intimidation and awe. "Wow!" she said "You have a *huge* angel!" I thought, *Oh, here we go!*

I was praying and feeling the whole thing out. I was a little baffled by God's leading on this one, and I began questioning my discernment. Not too far into the conversation she let me know that this session would cost $300. *Well! There's my answer!* I thought. I didn't have a dime to my name. I politely told her there was no way I could pay that, and trying hard not to offend her, I maneuvered my way out of the conversation and out the door as quickly as possible. Cynthia graciously followed my lead.

We got halfway to the elevator when we heard the apartment door open behind us. "Listen," she said as we turned back, "I really think you should do this, and because of the nature of your situation I am willing to do this for free." I paused and answered, "I'll think about it and let you know." I had narrowly escaped the pressure of deciding and was glad to know that I'd gotten out of it. However, I continued to feel that I was supposed to do it, and since she'd offer to do it for free, I finally gave in and called her to make the appointment for a session.

A strange and eye-opening event occurred that night. I was sound asleep in the middle of the night when I felt someone shake me. The shaking jarred me out of my sleep. I was immediately awake and in a state of awareness. In that state of immediate awareness, I felt my body still physically moving from the shaking. I rolled over expecting to find Cynthia standing there with some sort of urgent news. I saw no one, but I knew someone was or had been there. There was no doubt. That morning I told Cynthia about the strange experience.

In the conversation with the psychic healer and her roommate, we had agreed to take them both to a popular coffee house in town the next morning. We picked them up mid morning. A few minutes after they got in the car with us, the psychic healer said, "So Jill, did you see me last night?" I knew immediately that she was talking about the strange experience. "I came to you in meditation. Did you see me?" she asked again. I explained what I had experienced. She said, "Well, could you see what I was wearing? I always like to put on different outfits and see if people can describe them."

My head was reeling over the absurdity of what she had just said, and while I did not see her, much less what she was wearing, I knew that her "meditation" was no doubt connected to my experience. She had powers that were not to be ignored. Again, I questioned God. Again, I felt led to move forward with her.

My session with her was to last four hours. I couldn't imagine why it needed to be that long. My surgeries had not even lasted that long. But if I was understanding God's leading in this, I believed that the second of the two purposes for this jaunt in the journey was that He was about to impart more insight regarding this mysterious realm we call the dark side. This was nothing like the rebelliousness of caving in to the lure of fascination with the Ouija board. To the best of my knowledge, He was the one leading me into it this time. As out of character as it seemed, I was sure it was Him, and I was sure I was safe.

I did not enter this session with the somewhat arrogant and dismissive attitude that I'd often had at that point regarding this type of thing. Once I had made the decision to follow Christ, it was exhausting and seemed unnecessary to spend time delving into any other line of thinking. But I went in believing that God wanted to reveal something to me in it. I reminded myself that Christians tend to make "devils" of things outside of their own understanding. Followers of other belief systems equally believe in their doctrines and equally cherish their validity and virtue.

In studying other religions I had to gain this reverence for other belief systems, and to this day I remain willing to find out that my doctrine is wrong. I maintain the conviction that either truth is exclusive and will continue to make itself known, or the game is not fair enough to concern myself with. So, once again I went in open-minded.

We spent the first few hours sitting on the floor beside a bed near a window. The psychic healer was an aging, petite, tanned woman who walked and sat with a slight hunch. I hung on every word, waiting for revelation— revelation from God, that is. I was watching for what God had to show me in this. She began to talk about the extraterrestrial beings that had joined us in the room, including my huge angel. I pictured this big, beautiful creamy-white mist of an angel standing next to the characters from the Star Wars bar and had to hold back a disrespectful snicker.

The first two to three hours was set aside for a cohesive presentation of her belief system. She stopped at one point and said, "I can see that you are sniffing out the evil in this, but what you need to understand is that there is actually no such thing as evil. Evil is only a concept. If you go looking for it, you will find it, but it is simply in your head." Most of what she was explaining was difficult for me to fully esteem, and she could sense that. I did my best to adjust my respect level and continued listening.

She began to explain the concept of twelve dimensions and out-of-body experiences, and shared that she frequently practiced out-of-body travel. In the year before I was diagnosed, I'd had a strange experience that I was very curious about but hadn't ever brought it up to anyone. I was innocently praying for a girl who had a brain tumor and was told she had hours to live.

I had my eyes shut, and in the middle of the prayer it felt as if I had lifted up out of myself, and I had this sensation of flying. Everything suddenly went black in my mind. Then I saw a speck of light in this darkness. I wondered if I was somehow witnessing her "light at the end of the tunnel" experience. Then instantly I was seeing her lying in a hospital bed with her sister sitting beside her. It was as if I were hovering over them the way you sometimes do in dreams, except that I was wide awake! I began telling her to rest. "Rest in the Lord. Just rest," I would say over and over. Then I snapped out of it, ended the prayer, and as usual, shook it off as weird and moved on.

That cancer patient made a miraculous turn for the better and actually went home from the hospital the next day. That got my attention, but she died two months later, so it all seemed impossible to understand. She was at least able to say goodbye to her children, her husband, and her family. She was not a Christian before then, and I was hoping she had accepted the Lord before she died. I still didn't know what to make of out-of-body experiences, but I continued soaking in everything the psychic healer was presenting.

She began talking about chakras. I had looked into chakras off and on, because back when everyone was making fun of Shirley MacLaine, I happened to watch Oprah one day when she was on the show. She was in the middle of explaining chakras, and it caught my attention because she was explaining something that I used to talk about.

When I ran track in school I figured out that there were levels of nervousness that I would experience. If I felt a ball of nervousness below my belly button, I was in good shape. I assumed this was what people called "butterflies." As long as it stayed below the belly button, it was an energy that I could use to my advantage. However, sometimes the ball of nervousness seemed to climb. I could feel the next level right under the bottom tip of my sternum. This is where I would start to lose a little control of my nervous energy. The next level was in the center of my chest, and when the butterflies made it to that level I became weak in the legs and physically shaky. Next was the throat. When it got to that point, I felt completely stifled.

This could also spark an asthma attack. I had to learn how to contain an asthma attack to keep it from intensifying.

I eventually learned how to focus and keep the nervous energy from climbing. These were the exact places on the body she was calling chakras. I decided Shirley MacLaine had gotten a bad rap for no reason. Eventually, I ran across the video version of her book. I rented it, but after watching it, it seemed like this enormous thing I'd have to tackle in order to get settled with. So again, I filed it under "weird" and went on. But now I was tuned in to the theory with heightened interest.

Then the psychic healer told me about planetary travel and how these beings in the room with us had traveled here from other realms and other planets, and how she too travels in that way. She referred to it as "the party on the planes." I pictured quantum leap planet-hopping, and if it were really possible, it would be a blast. I've always wanted to be an astronaut. Who needed a rocket if you could really do this? Earth, she explained, is the envy of all the cosmos. Everyone wants to be here in this dimension. That was a little confusing, because her roommate kept talking about how ready she was for everyone to move into the fourth dimension, which is what Christians call heaven.

For a brief period in my early 20s I became very curious about the Roswell account. The matching stories of seemingly unassuming people in that incident became fairly convincing to me. I was a mastering engineer for a while in Nashville, and I worked on a project that was the fourth album in a series from this artist. He offered to let me take the first three albums home and listen to them. I put the first one on and had an awful feeling come over me. I never remember being affected by music in that way. I had to turn it off. When I returned them he explained that the songs were written about an experience he'd had as a child. He, along with his entire family, totally believed they experienced alien abduction.

Another time in the mastering studio I was walking down a hall. We had a two-inch analog tape machine that we wheeled from studio to studio. It was sitting in the hallway. When I moved to get around it, I felt a shock wave go through me, and I involuntarily jerked my arm away from the machine. I looked down, bewildered, and Randy Kling, the owner, said, "Know what that is?" I said "No. What?" He pointed to the analog tape box sitting on top of the machine. "That is the original tape recording of John Lennon saying the Beatles were more famous than Jesus."

We did restoration work on analog tape for the Smithsonian Institute. I assumed that was why we had it. This shock wave seemed to be a supernatural jolt that went through me to warn me or give me a heads up. The jolt intrigued me more than the fact that we had possession of this famous master recording.

When the television show *Unsolved Mysteries* first started airing, I didn't miss an episode. Unless a person was actually confronted with such a bizarre happening, though, it seemed that people looked upon phenomena as mere entertainment, so that was how I chose to treat it. Sometimes when I'd think about it, it seemed amazing to me how passive everyone was about the evidence of such vast mysteries. The whole world just keeps pouring their coffee and running their vacuum cleaners.

The healer told me that I was going to have a spiritual graduation that few people ever encounter. They would go to what Christians perceive to be heaven, but I was destined to go to a higher place than that.

She talked about Christ consciousness, which suggests that Jesus was simply a teacher or messenger and a "master yogi" rather than the literal Son of God and actual part of the Godhead, as Christians believe. Jesus was merely a man who was unfailing in continuously tapping into the Christ consciousness. That consciousness is perfect wisdom, perfect love, and perfection itself. It was not God the Father that Jesus was tapping into. Jesus, too, was a time traveler like the psychic healer. This was how He walked through walls and walked on water. He was able to master the three-dimensional material realm, the world we know.

Finally, it was time to move from the classroom to a one-hour massage. Massage is something that people with intimacy issues have a hard time with. One, it is difficult to let your protective guard down enough to make it worthwhile, and two, it is hard and uncomfortable to perceive yourself worthy of such a fostering act of kindness. However, people had encouraged me to get massage therapy after the diagnosis. When I quit smoking, I decided to get a weekly massage with the money I was saving by not smoking. It helped motivate me to stick to my guns. So, I was looking forward to this part.

Once she began, though, it felt as if she was lightly poking me with something. With a tone of pride in her voice she said, "That is a gift I have. Does it feel like I have blades on the ends of my fingers?" For a second a fear came over me, and I pictured her having the long, gnarly fingernails of a witch—or worse, Freddy Krueger hands. I quickly found that silly and leaned back into God and dropped the fear.

She was laying different-sized crystals along my spine. She spent a bit of time focusing on the area of the tumor and proudly told me that she watched it lift and drift away from my body and into outer space. She had assured me this would work like surgery but in the cosmic realm rather than the material realm.

Then the fun part started. She began encouraging me to visualize some things and tell her what I saw. I thought it was a bit silly, but I am a creative person who has never found a blank screen in her head. I envy people who claim they do. I could easily let myself rummage through my thoughts and spew out some visuals to appease her.

I was getting tired and ready to move to the one thing I was really there for, which apparently would be the last thing on the agenda. She told me that our cosmic friends had followed us to the massage table, and even more had joined us. She sounded intrigued when she told me that they were terribly interested in what was happening there. My ego loves an audience, I guess, so I perked up a bit.

I remember seeing blue neon and not knowing why, but immediately presuming it was Atlantis. I didn't really even know what Atlantis was, but that is what popped into my head. Then I saw a tiny cupid-looking angel fly in toward me presenting a book covered in gold. The cupid opened the book and revealed its pink blank pages. She was happily handing it to me to keep. That one came from out of nowhere, and as creative as I may have ever been, I didn't normally have entire events play out in my head like that. It didn't cause alarm. I just assumed it was because I felt a pressure and desire to deliver, and therefore, I must have gone into some sort of hyper-creative mode.

She took me through an exercise that involved bringing my male energy and female energy into balance. That was going to be good for me, because more than one girl I knew had jokingly stated that if I lived with them, they wouldn't need a husband. I wasn't gay, just efficient. I was hoping I'd like to wear dresses more when I came out of there. It felt as if time was surely running out, so I reminded her of the forgiveness exercise.

It was evident that she had forgotten and didn't even feel it was significant, so she left me on my own. She encouraged me to do it the way the book had described. So to the best of my ability I visualized sitting by a campfire with my mom. I was sitting on one log, and she was sitting on another.

It was dark out. We were roasting marshmallows. I was supposed to visualize a relaxed scene. I had no idea how to really do this.

The psychic healer did eventually chime in. Right in the middle of my campfire scene she suggested that I dig up every little place of pain and find a hidden gift buried underneath. So my visual switched to that. I didn't know what kind of gift I was supposed to be finding. I was visualizing small, gift-wrapped boxes that I was digging out of dirt. I realized that couldn't be right, because the gifts were supposed to be under something, some pain. *What?* I wondered. Frustrated, I gave up on the visual exercise and silently cried out to God, *Oh, God, I just want to release my mother. Show me what to do.* It was a desperation that was coming from my heart of hearts. At a standstill in my spirit, I just waited and waited and waited, emotionally swimming inside a silent and deep desire to release her. I wasn't sure that I had accomplished anything but I had given it my whole heart. I was ready to come out from under the veil of this experience and go home.

It ended with that, and I politely thanked her for her hard work. I left the building and got into my car. It was dark outside by then, which made the session seem all that much longer. The minute I shut the car door, my cell phone rang. It was Mom. She hates talking on the phone and rarely ever calls anyone.

We talked for a minute, and I finally probed a bit by asking her what she was doing. She said, "Well, I've been reading the Bible, and God really struck me with the verse that says He has taken our sins and thrown them to the bottom of the sea. So, I'm just sitting here wondering that if my sins are at the bottom of the stinking ocean, then why in the world do I not just let go of all of my guilt?" I couldn't believe my ears. She never talked like that. It had to be connected with my moment of releasing her. It was at the very least God's way of letting me know that He acknowledged my heartfelt desire to release her.

I pulled out onto I-440 and headed back to Cynthia's. I could never drive that loop without thinking of the first time I came to Nashville. The brightest full moon I've ever seen shined a spotlight on Liz and me as we drove in the tunnel of trees along I-40. Nashville would eventually prescribe a classic love/hate friendship between us.

Liz and I met in Texas. At the time, Liz was married to Johnny Rose, the third in the trio with my husband and me. Liz struck me as a yuppie housewife, raising a teenage son and two beautiful baby girls. Liz had an amazing ear for a hit song and a budding curiosity about being a songwriter. At every turn the guys blew off her feeble efforts to join in the fun. I had learned every trick in the book for dealing with band members' wives. Rule number one: Befriend, like it or not!

Liz Rose was a force to be reckoned with from minute one. There was a mayhem that hung in the air over her that felt as if it required kid gloves. I was in the depths of grief over losing my brother at the time. I didn't have the energy for walking on eggshells. After the first night Johnny invited us for dinner, we weren't out of their driveway yet before I said, "I'm not going to be able to deal with that woman!" But I had a gut feeling she was supremely perched in my life, and I would just have to learn to deal with it.

Liz and I quickly found common ground though, through our taste for tequila and shared heartaches. As time passed and stories unfolded, I connected with Liz like no one I had ever connected with before or since. There was a hurting and locked-up little girl inside Liz too, and while I couldn't see that in myself at the time, I wanted her freed, and I decided it was my job to find the key. Music was that key. Liz saw the same hurt in me and knew music was my sanctuary.

My mother had pushed me to study copyright and publishing law from the time I was 15. I had acquired a small library of legal and educational books on the subjects. I encouraged Liz to study up on publishing as well and offered her the books. From what I understood about the world of publishing, I was convinced she would make a great publisher.

We all planned to move to Nashville, as soon as the time and money were right. We co-wrote her first song in the car, moving out to Nashville. I think we threw it away, but it was a victorious and liberating moment! We eventually opened a little publishing company on Music Row. Wanting to be perceived as a writer rather than a publisher, I was the "silent" manager of money during the initial set up phase. I moved on after getting signed to an artist/publishing deal with Milsap Galbraith Music Group.

Liz was different from me. She seemed to light up and love everything about Nashville and life on Music Row. For me, life on Music Row felt more like a huge traffic jam that I had to patiently pass through before I could get where I was going. I had a blast, though, because you just couldn't help it. The country music boom had turned that town into a perpetual party. It was electric back then. Liz is one of the most magnetic people I've ever been around. There was never a dull moment with us, and we kept those poor husbands of ours hopping. We were hanging out and becoming personal friends with country music superstars, drinking five hundred dollar bottles of Champagne, and playing the game. You couldn't hang around Liz and not have a blast. Our husbands spent many nights wondering if the two of us would turn up alive. We were Patsy Cline and

Loretta Lynn all over again, and we often went by "Patsy and Loretta."

After several months of scrounging around town trying to find our way to our own success, I got a phone call from a mutual friend of ours. She worked for a major record label. She told me a story of a backstabbing political move Liz had made on Music Row. I presumed it was true, and it cut me to the bone. It hit that unhealed wound of betrayal from childhood, but this time someone was messing with my only hope for Slone and me, the lottery of the music business. I shut her out and abandoned ship. She was left to try to understand what had just happened. I hardly gave her the time of day, much less an explanation of why I was so upset.

Months passed, and we began to try to patch things up, but by then Liz and Johnny were on the brink of divorce. In a failed attempt to play God, I decided to take it upon myself to fix the marriage. Uninvited, I swooped in, wearing my self-issued "superman cape" and overstepped my bounds. Through one issue after another between the two of us, we eventually just stopped staying in touch.

A year ago I was looking at a music business email. One of those flashing side advertisements that I hate was distracting me, so I moved to scroll it out of view. I glanced at it and saw that it was a picture of Liz. In a very important prayer the year before, I was listing things that I wanted in the next season of my life. On my list was the restoration of lost friendships. There wasn't a week that went by that I didn't miss and pray for Liz. Sometimes relationships are too unhealthy to be restored, and distance sadly remains necessary. So, I asked God to guide me in who I should attempt to restore friendships with. I was convinced the flashing picture was a green light from God.

I clicked the picture and watched a video of Liz accepting the Songwriter of the Year award. I bawled my eyes out watching her. I don't know that I've ever been more inspired by and proud of another person's accomplishment. As she cried in humbleness and gratitude for the enormous opportunity the community of songwriters in Nashville had given her, I saw that locked-up little girl in a rush of victory and I knew I had to call her.

I went out to Nashville on business not long after and spent the week with Liz. We sorted back through the details. Over a bottle of wine, we laughed and cried, and we buried that hatchet. I went to bed. I opened my Bible, and my eyes fell right on this verse: "Be kind to one another, tender hearted, forgiving one another, as God in Christ forgave you" (Ephesians 4:32 NKJV). Liz is quite possibly the most forgiving person I've ever met. My atheist friend used to say. "You've got too much hate in your heart, Jill." In my bitterness, I had been unable to be truly tenderhearted and forgiving. I was sorry so much time had gone by.

At one point after parting ways with Liz years ago, I remember realizing that I had lost the ability to trust and the ability to stay on top of forgiveness and, most importantly, the ability to truly love people. I loved to love people. I wanted that ability back. I was losing myself. At the time, my answering machine played the Sheryl Crow lyric, "Hello. It's me. I'm not at home. If you're trying to reach me, leave me ALONE!" Liz had earned her own hook of hatred there next to my mom's. Every little disappointment in Nashville then hung on Liz's hook.

Neither Liz nor my mother deserved the sentence of all the blame and resentment I was pinning on them. On the long walks I had been taking, I was letting go of fear and control and letting God take me down memory lane. I was learning that it is impossible to truly forgive without revisiting some things. He was taking things off the hooks one by one and sorting them out for me. He was revealing things that blew my mind and explained so much about how I had become who I had become. He was revealing lies that I had bought into along the way, lies that told me I was unworthy, and He was replacing the lies with the truth of who I was. He stood before me as a mirror, and the reflection was a version of me I didn't recognize.

He was revealing my bitterness and resentment as ugly sin. It was like an unattractive skin that I had been living in, but underneath it there was hidden beauty. It was the kind of beauty I had never felt worthy of having. I knew I would not shed the skin of bitterness and resentment overnight. He promised and proved to be a romantic who would walk with me through a process of coming into that real beauty. It would be years before I really began to see that promised beauty surface, but He gave me enough of a glimpse during those long walks to create a desperate desire to stay on that path with Him.

A few weeks had passed, and it was time to go back to Texas. I had stayed too long already. Cassie and I had booked a show on 9/9/99. It was the big Y2K scare day, and we thought we'd celebrate the world's survival that night, if we in fact survived it. We had booked the gig around a scheduled follow-up appointment with the oncologist. I had to fly out a week early due to that pain I was having. Since we'd discovered the mass, I was staying out there until I decided what to do next.

At the gig that night I came off stage and was waved down by a familiar face that I couldn't put a name to. She was complimenting me on the show, when it dawned on me that she was the "muscle-test girl" from the restaurant that night. I'd been wondering about her. I was also looking heavily into natural medicine and nutrition. Vaughan Penn was an angel in encouraging me in this. She threw a party and cooked organic foods, gave me a crash course, and set me on the right track. I had become a teetotaller in the all-important area of diet. I didn't know much about the mystery muscle-test girl, but I figured she was chock full of information on holistic medicine, and I wanted to pick her brain.

I stopped her in mid sentence and began to explain my story. She said, "Yes, I know your situation, and I've been waiting for you to come to me. I don't go to people; I wait for them to come to me." I was puzzled by what she said. "I've got to go out of town tomorrow," she said with urgency in her voice "I will be back in a couple of weeks. I will call you as soon as I am back in town. We need to get together. I'll explain then." I agreed, not sure what to make of the conversation.

A couple of weeks later Cassie threw a birthday party for me before I had to go back to Texas. It was rare that all the girls of The Gang were in town at the same time. This night almost every one of us was there. It was a great birthday gift and as I surveyed the room, I was reminded of how much I loved these women and how important they were in this journey.

We somehow all wound up sitting in a big square in the living room. JK had been talking about how we had always believed there was a reason that particular groups of people cross paths and connect. We all agreed there was some purpose for this circle of friends as well. In the spirit of the moment, completely out of character for any party The Gang had ever thrown, someone suggested that we say a prayer. We all scooted in and grabbed each others' hands. I was sitting next to Cassie. JK said, "Left hand up, right hand down." We all followed orders. Cassie looked at me puzzled and asked, "Do you feel that?" Wide-eyed, I said, "Yes!"

There was a surge of power pulsating between our hands. We let go. Everyone looked at us as we explained it. We smiled and shrugged our shoulders and re-locked hands.

Calina brought a friend named Jenn whom I had met at Van's Bible study. JK asked her if she would be the one to pray. "Would you pray one of those sweet prayers you pray?" she asked. I wasn't sure where JK even knew this girl from, but Jenn agreed. We bowed our heads, and she prayed, "Thank You, Lord, for being in this room with us. That power that Jill and Cassie feel is the power of Your Holy Spirit, and we thank You for it." She went on and prayed for this wonderful group of girls.

A few minutes after the prayer ended, the muscle-test girl showed up at the door. I didn't know she was back in town, and I didn't know who invited her. I was still sitting in the living room, and she came and sat next to me. She asked how I was doing, and I told her I was hanging in there. I told her I was headed back to Texas the next day. She seemed to be trying to hide her anxiousness.

Cassie had some amazing pieces of art in her house. Earlier in the night I noticed a piece I'd never seen before. It was a gold-plated short wand of sorts with a purple crystal ball on the top end. I was holding it in my hand. I had become very curious about crystals, as well as other stones, and the belief that they contain healing elements. Cassie bought me some healing bead bracelets, and I began wearing them all the time.

This girl finally leaned in and said, "You, you…if you're going to carry that wand around, you might want to cleanse it with some sea salt and olive oil." She told me that she'd heard I had visited the psychic healer, and she tactfully warned me to be careful. She explained that she was going to go meet with her the next day, not as a client, but as a peer. I was not sure exactly what she was implying. Then she said, "Do you mind if I...?" as she leaned in and touched my knee.

I was getting used to these spiritual types. I had been at a party not long before. A spiritual guest randomly put her hand lightly on my shoulder and said, "You like carbs, don't you? You love potatoes because you need rest and comfort." It reminded me of a time when I was in my early 20s. I was at a corporate Thanksgiving dinner and mentioned that I don't like chicken and dumplings because I don't like soggy bread. A woman I'd never met in my life who was sitting at the next table said, "Do you stir your ice cream and let it melt a bit before you eat it?" I said, "Yeah. How did you know that?" She said, "You're a Libra, aren't you?" I am.

When the girl touched my knee she said, "I'm sorry to do this, but this feels like an emergency. Is there any way we could go in Cassie's bedroom?" I was starting to feel that there was no coincidence to the timing of all these people on and off of my path. They were like pawns atop a spirit-realm chessboard. "Sure," I said and stood up to lead her to Cassie's room. We shut the door behind us.

She asked me to lie back on the bed in a comfortable position. She got on her knees and brought her hands to prayer position against her mouth. She sat silent for a few seconds. Then, she stood up and put her hand first on my elbows and then on my shoulder the way a doctor would if he was examining a sprain. She said to herself but aloud, as if she was making verbal notes, "Oh wow! There is a mother, and there are sisters and ... listen. You cannot go back to Texas tomorrow. You won't survive."

I was trying to imagine what she was seeing in her invisible crystal ball. And I was trying to get a grip on the urgency in her voice. Then she let her hand hover over that chakra at the bottom of the sternum. I immediately felt an intense heat penetrate straight through me. A reflex caused me to shoot up in sitting position, and I let out an involuntary, moaning cry. Tears flowed uncontrollably. The girl backed up with wide eyes and said, "Whoa! …That's … good. That's really good." It was obvious she had impressed herself.

It all happened so fast I didn't have time to think about it. JK walked in on her way to the bathroom, and in the heat of the moment the girl abruptly asked her to leave. "We are in the middle of something here," she said. JK stepped out.

She then talked me through a thirty-minute process of revisiting different ages in my life. She would ask me to tell her about events from my first-grade year and questions of that nature that would spark a visceral effect, so that I could get in touch with the things from different periods of my life that were still burdening me.

While it was interesting and God seemed to be further revealing things, I had a hard time giving it my full attention. I was concerned about making the call to Texas to tell my family I was not coming back yet. I was flying on my dad's frequent-flyer miles so I could easily change the tickets, but I could feel in my bones that they were beginning to be very upset with me for leaving Slone with Rona. I did not explain everything to them. I had written a detailed email telling the family that I was refusing the surgery, but I was not keeping them informed of the details of those couple of weeks. It looked to them as if I was just partying, and I knew they probably assumed I was neglecting Slone to be with my new boyfriend in Nashville. The truth was that I rarely saw Jim during that month. I spent most of it alone.

I made the call. As crazy as it may have sounded, I was alarmed by the warning that I would not survive. I was not taking any chances, because I believed that every step was being led by God. I had never been so surrendered and obedient in my life. If God did not honor that by leading me not into temptation and delivering me from evil, then what chance did I have at anything? I spent another week walking, watching, and listening. In that week I became convinced that I had to finally talk face-to-face with my mom about the past.

God had highlighted the passage from Ephesians for me that says "For we do not wrestle against flesh and blood, but against powers and principalities, against rulers and authorities, against the spiritual forces of evil in the heavenly realms" (Ephesians 6:12 NIV).

I had to realize that my mom could not be to blame, fully. The battle was not between me and my mom. It was not between me and the abuser. It was not between me and the rapist. The influence of sexual perversion, which seemed to certainly be a spiritual force of evil had entered our lives and wrecked these relationships. I saw that my mother and I needed to lock arms and stand against the forces of evil together, in Christ, from that point on!

I rehearsed in my head and in my heart what I would say and how I would say it. This was something that had needed to be confronted for so long, but there was never a good time to do so. There was never going to be a good time in life to do this. I knew the chances of it going smoothly were very slim. In my family, the girls are not made of sugar and spice and everything nice. In our brokenness, we are made of jagged edges and open wounds. If you get us too close together, we cannot keep from hurting each other.

I knew what I wanted to say. The first time I was sexually abused was sometime before I entered first grade. I must have been 5 years old. The "evil force" was clearly ruthless. Somewhere along the way I had picked up a shield and dagger of distrust, and it stood between me and everyone I ever came in contact with. I knew that the last two people on earth the shield and dagger should be between were my mother and me. I would explain that to her, and I would lay them down once and for all.

In order to get over the mountain of hurt, I felt I would have to muster up the guts to finally talk to her about the conversation we had when I was 14 that brought about my hatred for her. I also knew that I had to drive back to the panhandle of Texas where I grew up. It seemed important to physically revisit some places in the process of letting go of the past.

Once I got back to Texas, Stacy affirmed my suspicions about how the family was feeling about my time in Nashville. I was feeling dreadfully misunderstood, and I didn't even know where to begin in explaining it all. She also lovingly confronted me about the healing beads I was wearing. She had been supportive of the little she knew about my journey in walking away from the surgery, but she felt she had to draw a line and let me know she did not believe in depending on material things such as these beads. I justified wearing them by explaining to her that I was not so convinced of their power to heal, but for me it represented the life-giving love and support that my friends in Nashville had shown. She said that she could understand and appreciate that. She invited me to go to church with her later in the week.

I planned to talk with Mom, go to church with Stacy at the end of the week, and then drive to the Panhandle. Mom and I met at Rona's, but for lack of privacy we left and drove around to talk. I was prepared to carefully pass through this delicate china closet, but I quickly became a nervous and clumsy bull inside. I said the things I had rehearsed, but still, I cut like a knife.

She tried to be the gracious mother, letting her daughter vent, but this was more than she could take. I was being relentlessly selfish this time, and I felt I had to take the burden of the misplaced shame and blame from that painful conversation off my back and lay it at her feet. I had to say, "I was not the one to blame. This shame does not belong to me, and I have to rid myself of it." I felt my life depended on it this time.

I was walking around with this mass as if it were a deadly spider on my shoulder that had to be carefully and precisely knocked off. I was scared of dying. I wanted us to come out of that conversation hugging in triumph, but it did not happen. What was done was done, and I felt I had to keep moving.

Rona was working for a former employer of mine. I had come through Dallas for a short time before moving on to Nashville. When I left for Nashville, she took over my position. She asked me to come in and see her boss before I drove to the Panhandle. I agreed.

He led me to a private area of his offices and sat me down. I had never seen him so serious. He was fighting back tears as he begged me to get my head on straight and stop messing around and have this surgery. He told me of friends of his that had gone through similar surgeries and how it had prolonged their lives. "You've just *got* to do this, Jill!" he pleaded.

I was stifled by the burden of all the misunderstanding, and it was clear there would be no understanding, no matter how hard I tried to explain what I had been going through. I could read between the lines, and it became evident that Rona was in total agreement with his opinion.

Even a few members of The Gang had gotten together over dinner during my time in Nashville to discuss my decision. One of the girls was not in agreement with my decision. I wasn't told which one, but word got back to me that she actually said, "Jill is playing games with her son's mother's life!"

I left the office, and in my car these comments began swarming me. I wept in fear that I had been such a fool to lean on the support and advice of my illogical, ethereal songwriter friends in Nashville. It seemed so unfair that God would allow me to be so deceived. *Why are You putting me through all of this chaos? Is this You or not?* I shouted. I had to know the status of this mass as soon as possible. I decided to visit a chiropractor in Arlington that I'd met. She sold a supplement I was taking. She could prescribe a sonogram, so I asked her to set up an appointment for the procedure for the following week. I wasn't ready for the chastising I knew would come from the oncologist when I tried to explain myself.

I had time to go back to the Panhandle before the appointment. I kept my commitment to go to church with Stacy before leaving. I had been reading the book Calina had given me, *Love, Medicine and Miracles*, the night before. I was thinking about it in the car on the way to church. In the book, the author, Dr. Bernie Siegel explains that he came to know and develop a relationship with what he believes is his personal spirit guide. He calls him George. Seeking an explanation, a woman is referred to Dr. Siegel. She describes a white-robed male who is always present with her. As I thought about it again, a passion rose up in me, and I knew in that moment that I had to tell people the story of the night of my diagnosis. The "white-robed male" who had manifested himself to me that night was Jesus! He was none other than Jesus, and people had to know that.

After being anointed once again with oil by some of Stacy's friends who prayed a powerful prayer for healing, I observed the rowdy conduct within this peculiar congregation from my aisle seat. I had never seen the likes of these Christians. This was apparently what a "move of the Holy Spirit" looked like. I wondered how they could have anything against spiritualism, mysticism and the like, when they were wildly rolling around and radically rocking back and forth down on their knees in worship. It was fanatical!

I was feeling a little defensive about my own journey and wondering what the real difference was in all this whacky spiritual stuff. Then in the midst of all this fanaticism, the most humble, down-to-earth, and mild-mannered preacher took the pulpit. He looked to be in his sixties and he seemed as level-headed as my favorite preacher, Gerald Mann. His name was Doug White and he seemed to be quite a dichotomy in this environment. It convinced me that whatever was going on here was out of his control and authentic. It seemed that he, like me, was clearly doing his best in letting God have His way. If this man could put up with the wildness of what I was witnessing, then I didn't need to feel foolish or bad about my efforts to follow that same God in my own journey.

Fire

I drove to the Panhandle in the quietness of night. I would break that silence to my own surprise. Something seemed to be stirring in me and I suddenly burst into shouting prayer inside my car. I had never prayed like this but, I believed in Satan, and with a vengeance, I began claiming my life back! As I prayed, I began to have visions of small fires all across the acreage of the county I was raised in. "You have stolen my life, Satan, but I am here to take it back!" I shouted. I was shocked at myself, but I went with the fervor, and when I was done I was free!

I spent the weekend with my precious grandparents. They were the solid rock of our lives when we were growing up, and their house was a haven. It was the perfect landing place to regroup before going back to Arlington. Before I left, I revisited some places. I went back to the site of the rape. I drove past houses I had lived in.

I prayed for my perpetrators. I knew the hellish prison of being the victim, but it now seemed almost easy in comparison to the hellish prison of being a perpetrator. The way I saw it, they were the bigger victims. People take pity on a victim of abuse but have no mercy for the perpetrator in the way that Jesus does—and calls us to. They do not look through the lenses I was seeing through. They do not see this spiritual war we are in together, and too many stay locked behind the bars of the world's condemnation rather than finding liberty in Christ.

We must own our sin and come to true and sincere repentance for what we've chosen to fall into while we are under the influence of evil. I prayed that my perpetrators would surrender and find life and freedom in Christ. I was forgiving them in the same way that He was forgiving me for my sinful choices.

When I was kid there was a certain set of railroad tracks that I used to go to. We used to pull thin rusted metal pieces off the tracks. You could break them off, bend them in half and blow through them. It made a loud whistle. I wanted to find one and take it back with me. It would be my token reminder of this time of truly forgiving and letting the past go. I would frame it and hang it in my house. No one needed to know what it represented, but I would know.

When I reached the tracks I noticed that all of that metal has since been replaced. As I walked down the tracks I closed my eyes and prayed, "God, I know it's silly, but I really wanted something to take back with me. So would You show me something, a rock or something, that would be our little code keepsake." When I opened my eyes, I noticed a railroad spike at my feet. I picked it up and thought that it would be the perfect reminder of the railroad tracks. It wasn't a whistle, but it was railroad-related, and it would do.

As I drove the six-hour drive back, I decided to listen to the Bible on cassette tape. My mother had given each of her daughters a set. I put in the first book of the New Testament, Matthew. I listened to the entire book of Matthew. As I listened, an atmosphere of revelation filled my car. I began to see and hear the truth of the gospel of Jesus Christ in a whole new way. Razor-sharp clarity and discernment came to me as I thought about the experiences that God had paraded me through in this healing process. I had kept an open mind about many things as we walked this path. For example, the suggestion that crystals and certain other types of stones contained healing power. I believed that this could easily be true and that it is not even a stretch to believe so. If stones did have healing power though, it was only because the Creator placed properties that had the power to heal within the stones.

As I listened though, I became aware of the fine line of idolatry in my own heart. I was convicted as I realized that I actually had been placing at least a portion of my hope in the material things such as the beads that I was wearing or crystals. I would look at them and hope they were working somehow. I recognized that *all* of my hope had to be in the Healer and none of my hope could be in the means by which He chooses to heal me. While Jesus was on earth, He healed people in a variety of ways. One woman touched the hem of his garment and was healed. Jesus mixed his own spit with clay and healed a blind man with it. So many times I've relied entirely upon the word of doctors, or the reports of tests and the effects of medicine. I was recognizing that these were subtle forms of idolatry.

Since "The earth is the Lord's and everything in it, the world and all who are in it." (Psalm 24:1 NIV), I knew that He could choose to use any thing or any one to administer healing to me. But I was gaining new levels of conviction about the fact that Jesus is *the* Healer and the Healer *alone*, heals. I realized that I must put 100% of my hope in Him, the healer, and not in anything else, including doctors and medicine—even if He chose to use them. My hope had to be in the Healer. My focus had to remain on Him. When my hope and focus were turned to things and people, to some degree, I blocked my connection to God Almighty—my only source of life.

The issue of idolatry though, is a matter of the heart and can only be judged by God. As I listened to the book of Matthew, it was as if God's word took on a presence that filled the car and started judging my heart matter. By judging, I don't mean hitting me over the head with condemnation and shame. It was His Spirit, gently pointing this out, in a loving manner, for my own benefit. I didn't know it at the time but would later learn that the Bible actually says that out-right. In Hebrews 4:12 it says "For the word of God is living and active. Sharper than any double-edged sword, it penetrates even to dividing soul and spirit, joints and marrow; it judges the thoughts and attitudes of the heart" (NIV).

So, of all these things: crystals, psychic healers, healing beads, wheat grass, surgeries, herbal teas, diet, forgiveness exercises, long walks, memories, CAT scans, sonograms, tofu, angels and the idea of extraterrestrials, there was only one thing I needed and that one thing was the Healer. His word was washing over me as I listened. It was cleansing, renewing and freeing me from the residue of idolatry I had been walking in. It was clearing out the perplexity of all the things outside of Him that I had taken in and considered.

I heard the words of Jesus in the book of Matthew saying, "Enter through the narrow gate. For wide is the gate and broad is the road that leads to destruction, and many enter through it. But small is the gate and narrow is the road that leads to life and only a few find it" (Matthew 7:13-14 NIV).

I didn't know whether I was going to survive cancer and stay alive or "lose the battle" and die. All I knew was that I wanted to get on, and stay on the road that leads to the life

Jesus had talked about. I knew in that moment, that the decision to go after that life would cost me but I was finished with wrestling Him for my broad-road version of "life". I wanted His. There was not one thing I needed in the entire infinite universe outside of Jesus Christ.

In the Old Testament there is a story that seems bizarre at first. The story tells of an incident that happened while the Jewish people were in the desert. God had miraculously rescued them from brutal slavery in Egypt. He promised to lead them to a land where they would prosper and be safe as long as they would surrender to Him, listen to Him, and follow Him.

On their way to the Promised Land, God had led them into the desert. Some had become very impatient and rebelled against their leader, Moses, and against God. Poisonous snakes appeared and bit the people, and many of them died. The people came to Moses and admitted their sin of impatience, their lack of trust, and their rebellion. They asked Moses to pray and ask God to remove the snakes. God then gave Moses a strange instruction, telling him to "make a snake and put it up on a pole; anyone who is bitten can *look at it and live*" (Numbers 21:8 NIV—emphasis added).

In the New Testament this story is referred to, and its significance is revealed. "Just as Moses lifted up the snake in the desert, so the Son of Man must be lifted up that everyone who believes in him may have eternal life. For God so loved the world that he gave his only Son, that whoever believes in him shall not perish but have eternal life. For God did not send his Son into the world to condemn the world, but to save the world through him" (John 3:14–17 NIV).

As I was listening to the book of Matthew I was "looking at it" again. I had to consider it, ponder it, question the work on the cross, and again receive revelation concerning it. I now realize that through the book of Matthew, the Lord was saying to me, "Look at it and live!"

After years of opening myself to His correction and revelation, I have landed on the belief that God led me through, or at the very least allowed, these experiences with the psychic healer and the healing arts in much the same way that He led Daniel through or allowed the experience of being involved in the magical arts—and later even allowed him to be appointed chief of the magicians, enchanters, astrologers, and diviners.

To God's glory, at no time did Daniel worship the gods of these diviners as is chronicled in the book of Daniel. At no time was I ultimately seeking a medium, as is warned against in the Bible. I was seeking God Almighty, who was opening my eyes to the real power of divination. I had been paraded through a cast of characters possessing very real abilities to control and manipulate others. The reality that someone had the power, through meditation and the magical arts, to actually invade my life in the middle of the night while I slept, was an awakening!

After listening to the book of Matthew, I began stepping into the awareness of the real power and authority we have been given in Christ over such control and manipulation. The source of power in the magical arts is demonic. I came to know that I am called and commissioned to come out of my complacency and stop tolerating these powers and become a conqueror in Christ *over* these powers in my life as well as in the lives of others.

As I was pulling into Dad's driveway after arriving back in Arlington, Stacy met me at my car. She noticed the railroad spike and asked me what it was. I told her about it. She said it made her think of the verse in the Bible that talks about Christ nailing our sins to the cross. I hadn't even seen the significance of my forgiveness souvenir until she said that. I decided to find that verse after she left.

The passage is found in Colossians 2:13-14: "When you were dead in your sins, God made you alive with Christ. He forgave us all our sins, having canceled the written code that stood opposed to us, He took it away, nailing it to the cross. And having disarmed the powers and authorities, he made a public spectacle of them, triumphing over them by the cross" (NIV). It dawned on me that I had found that spike at my feet and that His work on the cross was Jesus, humbling Himself to come and serve at the feet of His people.

Dad, who was actually my step father, had adopted Rona and me when I was 2. Even though he and my mother divorced soon after that, he has taken care of us ever since as if we were his own. When he invited me to stay with him, he told me that he wanted his house to be a place of refuge for me, and it was.

My dad was someone who always seemed to understand me. I always knew I could count on him even with all my entangled trust issues—none of which he could have prevented. Even if I had found the guts to confide in him and tell him the secrets of my childhood, I'm not sure what he could have done about it all. I did finally divulge my secrets to him after returning from the Panhandle. I hoped I wasn't being selfish but I could not get over the burden that had lifted as a result of being secret-free after all those years.

A beautiful upright piano that had belonged to his mother and now belonged to Stacy was in the formal dining room of his house. I spent hours alone the next morning playing that piano in gratitude. When I had finished playing, I went to the living room and continued praying and marveling in the Lord, feeling completely free for the first time in my life.

Suddenly I realized I could see into the spirit realm as if it had meshed together with the structure of the living room. Heaven had opened up, and I could sense angels looking down at me. It was overwhelming, and I began to cry. Aware that my dad might pull into the driveway and walk in any moment, I was afraid of how he would react. So, I walked out of the living room and opened the door to the room I was staying in. The presence of the Lord was tangibly manifested again, and I was aware that He was sitting on the end of the bed. I collapsed into His lap and wept and wept and wept.

I wept in worship and as I did, emotional pain emptied out of me and into Him. I became aware that Jesus is the only being in existence that has the capacity to carry the burdens that this dark world imposes upon us. There is no other vessel capable of seizing it all. There is no other name by which we are saved than Jesus. There is no counselor, no passion, no person, no career, no addiction, nor obsession on earth that can retain all of our grief and anguish. Jesus can and will.

Fruits and Nuts

*I*t was now finally time to deal with this mass. Stacy went with me to the imaging center. An assistant called my name, and I could feel the regret building in my gut. I was afraid they would discover a basketball-sized mass, but no matter what the results were, I knew without a doubt that I was in Christ and He was in me. That was all that mattered to me. Stacy waited in the waiting room. The technician stared at the image, and I could see that the mass was still there as she measured it.

The two smaller almond-size masses were no longer attached. She looked alarmed, not knowing any of my history. I asked, "Can you tell me what size it is?" She said, "Oh, I really can't discuss that with you. Your doctor will go over the results with you." I said, "Well, look, I already know about the mass. I just needed to know the size of it." She looked perplexed and asked, "Why didn't you go to your doctor for this?" I didn't want to explain that. "It's a long story, but I can see the mass on the screen. Would you say it's the size of a lemon?" I probed with wishful thinking. She whispered, "No, more like the size of a walnut, but I really am not supposed to discuss this. I'll be right back."

A walnut, I thought *No way!* I couldn't believe it! It was going away! I wanted to dance! The doctor came in and told me she would release the scans to my chiropractor. She seemed to be a little put out with my scam. I was beaming when I came back into the waiting room, but I made Stacy wait for the news until I paid and we got out to the car.

The mass was 5 centimeters in diameter. There was a ruler in my day planner, and I was digging it out to look at it as I was telling her what had happened. I just couldn't get over it. We stopped at a grocery store on the way home because Stacy needed a few things. I stood in the produce aisle holding up a walnut in one hand next to an orange in the other. Another shopper looked at me as if I was crazy.

I rested for a few days in the peace and presence of the Lord. At times I would lie down on the bed and a visualization and feeling would suddenly come, as if I was lying in a gentle stream. The stream seemed to be sweeping over me, further healing me.

A man, believed to be John, had an encounter where he visualized incredible things. His vision is recorded in the book of the Bible called Revelation. In chapter 7, verses 9-17 he states he saw this: "After this I looked and there before me was a great multitude that no one could count, from every nation, tribe, people and language, standing before the throne and in front of the Lamb. They were wearing white robes and were holding palm branches in their hands. And they cried out in a loud voice: "Salvation belongs to our God, who sits on the throne, and to the Lamb." All the angels were standing around the throne and around the elders and the four living creatures. They fell down on their faces before the throne and worshiped God, saying: "Amen! Praise and glory and wisdom and thanks and honor and power and strength be to our God for ever and ever. Amen!" Then one of the elders asked me, "These in white robes—who are they, and where did they come from?" I answered, "Sir, you know." And he said, "These are they who have come out of the great tribulation; they have washed their robes and made them white in the blood of the Lamb. Therefore, they are before the throne of God and serve him day and night in his temple; and he who sits on the throne will spread his tent over them. Never again will they hunger; never again will they thirst. The sun will not beat upon them, nor any scorching heat. For the Lamb at the center of the throne will be their shepherd; he will lead them to springs of living water. And God will wipe away every tear from their eyes."

I soaked up the reality of the shrinking mass as I lay there in this stream of spirit realm "living water", and I knew what I was going to do. I was moving back to Nashville as soon as possible. I even called my apartment manager there and asked if I could have the very same apartment back. I wanted my life back, as if none of this had ever happened. I understood that the mass was not completely gone, but I knew what God had told me, and He was proving Himself faithful.

My apartment was taken, but an identical one in the next building was available. I took it sight unseen. Slone practically lived for basketball, and he had just started the season on an awesome team with a great coach. I decided to let Slone finish out the basketball season in Arlington before moving back with me. I was going back to find temp work until after the holidays. I would travel back and forth between Arlington and Nashville, and we would both officially move back in January.

I packed up my car and went to Rona's to say goodbye to Slone. I was walking out the door to leave when Rona's phone rang. She came out and said that mom was on the phone and wanted to say goodbye. I got on the phone, and we did what we do best. We acted as if nothing ever happened and kept it light and above the surface. Just before I hung up the phone I heard her say, "Jill." I put the receiver back to my ear and said, "Yeah?" She said, "I love you with all my heart." I melted. "I love you, too," I said, and we hung up. The power of those words was weightier than I'd ever imagined.

My mother has a beautiful heart. On this journey the Lord allowed me to begin seeing her for who she really is, not for what she had done. He made me see and accept that she, like me, has a story of burdens that have locked her up and shut her down. The Lord offered me the benefit of discovering video of her when she was a little girl. As I watched her beautiful blonde curls bounce and her beaming smile, I came to know her in a new way.

People had betrayed her and hurt her too. I realized that if we want to play the blame game, if we want to find one hook to hang the burden of responsibility upon, we will keep digging back, generation to generation, and wind up at Adam and Eve. We live in a fallen world, and people hurt other people here. I was called to forgive in the way that Jesus has forgiven me. The first time the Holy Spirit led me through the memory of that conversation with her when I was 14, it played out in my head exactly the way it played out in real life. It sparked the same feelings of abandonment and betrayal. These feelings would cause me to physically shake. But then the Lord pushed me to look at it again. This time I saw it play out as if I was a third-party witness, and for the first time I saw her side of that incredibly delicate situation. I understood why she handled it the way she did.

My step grandmother was the regional director in the Panhandle of Texas for Child Evangelism Fellowship. She spent her life teaching countless children about the love of

Christ. Without the seeds she planted in me, I'm not sure where I would be. She had passed away shortly before my diagnosis. We sang *Jesus Loves Me* at her funeral - a sweet and appropriate tribute to her work. I can not wait to wrap my arms around her in heaven and thank her.

I remember Jesus beckoning me back then. I asked him "into my heart" and was as sincere as a 9-year-old can be about being a Christian. That original conversation with Mom took about fifteen minutes, and roughly two pages of this book were used to describe that entire traumatic season. That season consumed years of my life. It took over twenty years of festering and decaying before I would take Jesus up on what He had offered me when I was 9 years old:

"Come to me, all you who are weary with heavy burdens, and I will give you rest. Take my yoke upon you and learn from me, for I am gentle and humble in heart, and you will find rest for your souls. For my yoke is easy and my burden is light"

(Matthew 11:28-30 NIV).

On one of my trips back to Texas, Rona gave me a devotional called *Streams in the Desert*. She wrote a note on the inside cover that included one of the most incredible poems I'd ever read. I was thinking about that poem days later, and I went back to see who the writer was. I wanted to find more of the poet's work. I read it again and realized Rona had written it.

I think about everything that has happened and I realize how proud I am of the women of my family. There is no point in this story where we are all brushed off and packaged up and standing in front of you wearing tiaras, blinding you with sparkling smiles, and waving our little white gloves, but we are a beauty to behold! Renewal is a daily affair, and we press on through the peaks and valleys of this life, together in Christ.

Home Again, Home Again, Jiggity Jig

*H*ome is where your heart is, they say. Nashville had simply become my home. I was back and couldn't be happier. I took a corporate job outside the music business. I was done with the Music Row phase of my life. I felt as if I had made it through that traffic jam and I was flying down the highway. I was eager to get back to Christ Church and dig deeper and deeper into the things of God.

I had recorded several guitar vocals at Jim's, and he had worked on them off and on, but we hadn't really gotten anywhere with them. I began feeling a strong tug in my spirit that the Lord was encouraging me to break the ties with Jim and allow myself to walk alone with Him. As I had gone through the process of revisiting the pain of my past, I began to feel a desperate grief over the loss of my virginity.

I did not know why that was so important to me. Almost every girl I've ever known willingly gave up her virginity before marriage. Something about the rape seemed to make me determined to get my virginity back on some level, and I began asking God if that was at all possible. I made a commitment to God to be single for two years. I couldn't see any way a woman could regain her virginity, but I knew that

I needed to be deprogrammed and reprogrammed where sex and men were concerned.

Stacy called me one day, and we were discussing these things. She said "You know, Jill, there is a story in the Bible about a girl who was raped, and it was pretty much swept under the carpet. I don't know the story all that well, and I can't remember where it is in the Bible, but you ought to find it."

The following Sunday I heard a quick reference in a sermon about this very story from the Bible. The preacher mentioned the rape victim's name was Tamar; the story was found in 2nd Samuel 13. I went home and got out the navy blue, silver-lined, thumb-tabbed NIV Study Bible that my mom bought me. I turned to the passage and read it. I wept again in the healing. It felt as if the story was included in the Bible just for me.

I wanted to be pure. I wanted to understand the desperate desire to be pure. I wanted to understand why rape affects a person in the way that it does. I wanted to know why those affects stayed with a person the way they did—why it seemed impossible to shake those affects.

I wanted to understand sex. I wanted to know God's true purpose, design and original objective for sex. Though it was hard to grasp and believe at first, the Holy Spirit began assuring me that I could "regain" virginity. He made me see that in a sense, I *was* a virgin. I had never even come close to experiencing the kind of sex that He designed. Sex is spiritual. I knew nothing about it. He would someday give me the chance to experience it but only after a process of patiently letting Him completely reprogram my mind and heart.

The following Wednesday I was waiting for church to begin, and I was reading the passage again, thanking God for all He had done. A girl sat next to me and started a conversation. I laid my Bible down beside me. She mentioned 2nd Samuel. I said, "Wow, I was just reading out of 2nd Samuel." I grabbed my Bible to show her, and as I dragged it across my lap, I noticed that the corner of the page I was reading was dog-eared. I quickly unfolded it in an effort to keep this gift from my mother pristine.

When I unfolded it, we could both see that the page had apparently been cut incorrectly. The dog-ear unfolded and stuck out above all the other pages. I folded it back down and noticed that it was shaped like an arrow—and it pointed directly to this story of Tamar. Of all the Bibles in the world, this was the one that the Lord led my mother to buy.

Six weeks had gone by since I'd had the sonogram in Arlington, and it was time to face the music. I called my oncologist and scheduled the dreaded appointment in which I would be forced to explain the yellow brick road I had been on. She was not the least bit interested. She wanted facts and immediately sent me down the hall to have a CAT scan. In a couple of intense hours, the results came back. The only remaining mass was now 2 centimeters, the size of a grape. I was elated. She was not impressed. "Jill," she said, "if you had come in here originally with a mass this size, we would have prescribed the very same surgery. It still needs to be done." I looked at her as if she had to be kidding but decided to be respectful and cooperative.

She ordered a sonogram and explained that she needed it in order to see the exact position of the mass more clearly. When her assistant called to set up the appointment for the sonogram, as God would have it, the imaging center said the office would be closed for two weeks due to renovations.

Two weeks later I stared at a mass-free screen and watched a technician try to figure out what was wrong with the machine. She was holding the original "orange-sized" scan in her left hand and moving the computer mouse around with her right. She went to get a doctor to come look at it. The doctor took a few seconds to search around and then said, "You can't find it because it's gone." *She said it! "It's gone."* It echoed in my mind, *"It's gone."* I called my friends and left the message on answering machines across town: "It's gone!" "It's goh hoooonuh!" "It is *GONE!*" To this day, I remain cancer-free.

I had continued going to Van's Bible study. The group was led by Van and Karen's good friend, Mark Chesshir. He had a very patient and gentle pace and the power of the Holy Spirit among that group was uncontainable at times. There were a couple of wise older men that sat behind the kitchen counter, overlooking the living room. They often launched into passionate theological debates that were both entertaining and deeply moving. One friend referred to them as the "Muppet Judges" and the visual stuck. I could learn more about God's word from the Muppet Judges in one night than I could in a whole year elsewhere. God began to bring new friendships with mature, godly woman like Karen and friendships with great new Christians like Laurie Kerr. We walked it out together. We saw miracle after miracle as a result of our prayers in that group. But then we lost Van. It was alarming and confusing for me at first. Van's cancer was a much more advanced type than mine, but still, I didn't understand.

I began feeling fear and a loss of faith. Then I met Steve Shima. Steve also went to Christ Church. He had a brain tumor return from two years prior. At Vanderbilt they had done a sonogram the night before the second surgery. During the surgery the sonogram was displayed on one screen above the operating table, and the live surgery was displayed on a monitor on the other side of the table. It was a complicated and intricate operation. Young doctors observed from a balcony above as the surgeon repeated the intense surgery.

Steve tells the story of the spiritual struggle he went through the previous night, shortly after having the sonogram. In a battle with Satan he proclaimed "No matter what, even if death comes, you will never come between me and my God!" When the surgeon had clearly cut down to the location of the tumor, seeing that it was not there, a doctor in the balcony whispered, "He's got the wrong patient." The surgeon remained unshaken. He knew that he had the right patient for certain because he could clearly see the markings of the prior surgery.

His story was an injection of faith for me, and I had to come to accept that God is sovereign and His ways are not our ways. Cancer is caused by all sorts of things. My story, in my opinion, is not about a tumor or mystery mass that disappeared. My story is about a burden that was miraculously lifted. My cancer was hatred, and my hatred had been healed.

After we had broken up, Jim Kimball called one day and asked if I would meet him at Lake Radnor. He made it clear that it was not going to be about pressuring me to rekindle the relationship. I agreed to meet him. As we walked around the lake, he carried a camera bag belonging to a new camera he had around his neck. He asked if we could sit down for a bit. He reached into the camera bag and pulled out a portable CD player and headphones. Handing them to me, he said, "I want you to listen to something." I put the headphones on and listened. It slowly dawned on me that he had fully tracked the guitar vocal songs that I had left with him months before.

He had even secretly recorded a new song I did live at the Bluebird Café called "Salvation." He explained that he and several musician friends, who had gotten behind him in the idea, had tracked the songs for me. He said that he did it because he wanted me to know that people actually do good things for other people.

Jim continued to work on the project and would occasionally call me to tell me that he was having powerful encounters at times while he was working with the recordings. Jim spent many hours poring over electric guitar parts and finished mixes of four of those tracked songs. They are absolutely beautiful.

My life resumed its course, and we never finished the remaining tracks. I had recently sat in the Wallace Chapel of my beloved home church, tucked in the hills of Old Hickory Boulevard. There I heard the voice of the Lord clearly say, "I'm calling you into the ministry." So, into the ministry I went.

We members of The Gang began, one by one, packing up and scattering ourselves across the country. I will forever thank God for my time in Nashville and those incredible women who walked this journey with me and supported me the way they did. Their love was like an IV that sustained me. I cherish those friendships. Since I started writing this book, the emails have continued to fly. The reunion has taken shape and is now set in stone.

Occasionally, a friend or relative asks me the question that can spark a thousand feelings in me: "When will you record new songs?" The answer is, "I do not know." Le Roy Parnell once said, "Fame is just something I have to put up with in order to hold on to the freedom to do what I love." When I went to visit Liz for the first time in years, I sat alone for a moment in her swanky little writer's room beside her swimming pool behind her house. I stared at wall after wall of gold and platinum records, which afford her that freedom.

I experienced the inevitable moment of questioning: "OK, God. Let's address the elephant in the room. I am sincerely thrilled for Liz as I look around at all this and know the unbeatable odds she's overcome to get here. But why is it God, that *I* got ripped up out of this thing that has beckoned me since I was a kid?"

Another friend who is having amazing songwriting success in Nashville is an elementary school classmate of mine named Rodney Clawson. When we were in kindergarten, Rodney found a wet match under a willow tree on the playground. His eyes lit up, and he told me he was going to set that tree on fire. I ran in and told the teacher, but she put me in the corner for tattling on him. I stood in that corner for about thirty seconds and then quietly walked out the back door and down the alley to my house. I was called "The Kindergarten Dropout" from then on. To this day, I blame Rodney Dale Clawson for my inability to spell.

Rodney and I wrote together a little when he first started kicking around Nashville, but he called one day, got the Sheryl Crow answering machine message, and in my social dysfunction, I never returned his calls. I got a good chewing-out over that from one of our mutual school friends, and Rodney went on to get his walls filled as well. Rodney was a farmer writing songs from his tractor.

When folks back home first started telling me Rodney was trying to write songs, I didn't think anyone was taking him very seriously. This year Rodney is up for a Grammy for writing, in my opinion, the best song that has ever come out of mainstream country. The song is called "I Saw God Today." I heard a sermon once on the idea of what might have happened had Moses ignored the burning bush. As Rodney preaches in this song, we will see God if we look.

This is what I know. I would not trade a second of this journey for anything. The Bible says, "The one who finds his life will lose it, and the one who loses his life because of me will find it." I continue to do my best to follow hard after God's will for my life, and it has been a terrific ride so far. A songwriter was never something I wanted to be. It is something that I wake up and find I still am. Songs write themselves in me. I leave the rest to God. For now, "This is my story! *This* is my song!"

...and this is how it ends.

Time in the Sun

The Lord has never made Himself manifest in the way that He did the night of the diagnosis or that day on the end of the bed, but I have had countless incredible encounters with the Holy Spirit and the wonders of the heavenly realm since. I have daubed countless heads with oil myself now, and occasionally you will even find me radically "rocking and rolling" in worship. There is not a high in the world that can compare with being moved by the power of the presence of the King of Kings and Lord of Lords.

I fulfilled my commitment to spend two years single and set apart from the world I had known. At the end of the two years I could not imagine allowing anyone to interrupt my romance with God. He was my intimate friend, my sounding board, my prince of peace, my constant companion, my provider, and my king. I went into full-time ministry in various forms, and I loved my life. I remained single for seven years. Seven, in the Bible, represents completion. Eight represents new beginnings.

One Sunday, two years ago, I stood in church in Fort Worth, Texas, where I was living. I felt the presence of the Lord as if He had approached me. I could not see Him, but

I felt Him standing in front of me. Somehow, I immediately knew what He was there to say. I began to cry. I felt like a senior who was ready to graduate but afraid to leave home. He was telling me it was time, and He clearly ministered this to me: "I am about to make Myself manifest in your life in the form of a husband. He will be My arms." I wept at the thought of such a gift and at the bittersweet thought of moving beyond what I'd had with Him alone in the past seven years.

I had been spending a little time with an old friend in order to work on a business plan. After a few meetings, things began to lean toward dating. I had to assume this was the person the Lord was talking about. I had gone back to work for the same company I had worked for before moving to Nashville. My friend Laura was now managing the offices and needed temporary help.

The following Monday, I happened to be staring at my computer screen and watched as a name I hadn't thought of in years popped up into my inbox. "Kirk Welch?" I said. Laura looked at me. "What are you talking about? Who is Kirk Welch?" "He was my first love," I answered, "and he just sent me an email. He's married, though, so I don't know what he is doing emailing me. I really hate when married men do this kind of thing!" She rounded the corner of the desk and said, "Well, just see what he wants."

He sent an email explaining that someone had recently sent him an article about me. The article was in a small-town, online newspaper. He had gone to my website and listened to the songs. He congratulated me and said he was proud that I was writing songs for all the right reasons now. "I know how to handle this," I said. I sent him a polite email that simply said, "Thanks for your kind words. I hope you and your family are doing well." I hoped he would take the subtle hint of rebuke and disappear.

In Kirk's senior year of high school, he and his friends got together and mutually decided to break up with their girlfriends so they could be free for their final year. The other guys were not in long-term relationships. Kirk went along with the plan and came out to the house one day to hold up his end of the deal. It crushed me. A few weeks later he came and apologized. He told me that he realized that what he had done was a mistake. He explained that he knew our dating relationship was deeper than the dating relationships that the other guys had. He apologized for his pettiness. But it was no use, because I had done what I was so used to doing by then. I had stuffed it all inside, sewn it up, and moved on.

On a hiatus from college, Kirk had a job on a ski slope in New Mexico where we had snow-skied almost every weekend together when we were dating. He got word that I was separated from my husband, and he talked a friend into taking his job. He moved back home to pursue me. Even though I was separated from Slone's father, I was still trying to make the marriage work and had to turn him down.

Months later he was back in college, and I was divorced. He pursued again. I don't know that I understand why I did this, but I believe it was because I felt ashamed and that I was too much of a mess. He was my friend, and I didn't want him to step into my chaotic world. I finally sat him down one day and said "Look, you have a chance to graduate from college, plan a marriage, plan children, and do things the right way." I urged him to move on so he could do those things, and he did.

Not long after I replied to his email I received a response. He apologized for not explaining that he was now divorced. He assured me he would not be stalking me, but now that the conversation had opened up he wanted to take the opportunity to ask some questions: Are you still writing music? Do you have any more children other than Slone? Are you remarried? How is life in ministry? I answered as quickly as I could, trying not to be rude but feeling I didn't have time for it.

He sent an email back. In response to my answers, he answered some of the same questions. He explained that his ex-wife had met a man from California and was about to marry him and move to Los Angeles. In order to be with his two children, he was moving there also.

Laura is my best friend. She is my daily accountability partner. I share everything with her. I kept Laura in the loop of all the emails, and she began giving me a hard time asking if it was going to be "door number one" or "door number two" between these two men who were suddenly in my life.

There was also another sudden email out of nowhere from a friend I hadn't talk to in years. She was thrilled to add a "door number three" to her shtick. I knew it wasn't going to be Kirk, because I had just moved back to Fort Worth with a huge new business plan in mind and was not about to move to California. He sent me pictures of his two beautiful children. The thought of the divorce broke my heart for them. Coming from a few years in youth ministry, I felt I had to at least take the time to encourage him.

We moved from emails to telephone conversations. I told him my story. I was certain it would ultimately cause this West Texas Baptist boy to run screaming from this "psychedelic" super-freak of a Jesus follower. He seemed to hang on every word. I told the story he'd never known about me. He knew there was nothing he could have done about it at the time, but he said it made him feel even worse about the petty break-up.

He was equally overjoyed at what the Lord had done in my life. He explained that through his divorce, he had come to a rock-bottom place of surrender and was fully leaning on the Lord for restoration. He told me of some powerful encounters he'd had with the Holy Spirit during his healing process. We finally hung up in the wee hours of the morning. I felt like weeping for him for some reason that I didn't understand, but I was way too sleepy for that. I had to get what little sleep I could before heading to work.

I called Laura to kill time through a Dallas traffic jam and told her the story. She stopped me in mid sentence and said, "Jill, I don't know why but I'm about to bawl over this." I said, "Wow! That is exactly how I felt, and I don't know why!" Laura had become as much of a psychedelic super freak as I was in recent years, and all we knew to do was pray for Kirk and his move to L.A.

It was nearing Christmas, and I had offered to drive out to the Panhandle to get Boompa. He was having some trouble with his eyesight. Granny had passed away the year before and I could not stand for Boompa to be alone. I would drive him back to Arlington to be with us through the holidays. I agreed to meet Kirk for lunch while I was back there. I was convinced the Lord wanted me to make him aware of something He had revealed to me along the way.

In a book called *Inviting God to Your Wedding*, the producer of *Touched By an Angel* put it best when she explained that by God's design, sex causes a "soul tie." It is designed to be like a magnetic force, for the purpose of keeping a man and a woman committed to each other. When people decide to break that commitment, it is as if two two by-fours that were once glued together have been ripped apart. There are pieces of one board still affixed to the other and vice versa. The Lord will take you through a process of cleansing yourself of those pieces if you will allow Him.

God opened my eyes to see that His design is for one man and one woman to unite under His covering for life. He made me see how this reflects, in the physical realm, the beautiful picture of Christ, the Bridegroom, united for eternity with His bride, the church. Two people are biologically designed to procreate and bring to life the offspring of their own. I came to understand how this reflects the bringing to life of God's children, the beloved people of this world – the offspring of His Life. Through this I began to see and believe how much God loves this world. He made me see and believe that this is a design like any other design, such as that of a car or machine. If we choose to maintain or handle this design by any other set of principles, eventually it will break down.

I felt the Lord wanted me to share this insight with Kirk, and that maybe Kirk needed to do this work for himself. I had been through different exercises you can do for this purpose and had taken many youth members through this process. I felt it was even possible that God needed to take me through it again concerning Kirk.

Kirk was a little different from the others on the list for a few reasons. He was that first true love. Kirk and I had definitely been tied by our intimate relationship and sexual bond in high school. Our society simply does not understand the power of the bonds of intimacy that are designed to be reserved for marriage only. I have urged teens, due to my experiences, to wake up to this fact.

I had even been plagued by a recurring dream about Kirk in my early adulthood, due to this bond. I would dream that we were married and were back in the house he lived in during high school. His sister and mother would be there with me in the dining room, talking and laughing. We had two preteen kids, and they would be in the living room sitting on the floor playing. Kirk was not there, but

I knew we were good together, and all was right with the world. I would wake up from that dream, and before I really knew what was happening I would be crying out of the realization that the dream was not true. It would cause me to feel terribly guilty because usually when I had this recurring dream, I would wake up crying and find my self in reality, next to another man.

I was willing to revisit this if that was what God was leading me to do. I felt Kirk was going to move on, eventually find a wife, and walk in the blessings of his new commitment to the Lord. I was assuming I was about to marry my business pal and move into a new phase of my life as well.

We met, and I could tell that he was hoping it would somehow miraculously lead us into riding off into the sunset. I shared my thoughts about what God might be up to concerning "soul ties," but he seemed determined to hold out for something more. I think to ease his disappointment, I kept telling more stories of intense spiritual encounters I'd had, hoping he'd finally be relieved to part ways and once again move on. He wasn't easily deterred, though.

The day was getting late, and we both had to get going. He was driving me back to my car when he said something that made it evident that he was on the verge of tears. Trying to suck it up, he continued. I couldn't hold back, and tears started to well up. "What is this?" I laughed. "Why are we crying?" He stopped trying to hold back "I don't know! I cried all the way over here. I don't know what it is," he said. "Well, we can't just drive down Main Street bawling!" I said, "Pull over!" We were laughing and crying at the same time.

He pulled over and parked. He looked at me and said, "I was just hoping to somehow make it all up to you, Jill." And with that I involuntarily fell into his arms and burst into tears. It hit me like a sweet punch to the gut. I was a little embarrassed at my lack of control. He reached behind his seat to pull out a gift he'd bought for me. I was shocked. I opened it, and something about it struck me as so special. It was just a simple inexpensive watch he'd found in a Christian bookstore, but there was something so special about it.

We eventually pulled ourselves together and headed for my car. I leaned on the only thing I know. I said, "Let's pray." We grabbed hands and bowed heads. We each asked the Lord to do whatever He chose with all of it. We completely gave the situation to Him.

As I drove back to my granddad's house, I cried and prayed, *I don't know what that was all about, but I did it, God. I will let go of him now.* I was puzzled by my feelings. I wasn't holding on to him, that I knew of. I hadn't even thought of him in that way in years! I couldn't understand for the life of me why this was affecting me this way. But then, sometime in the middle of the night, I sat up in bed and said to myself, "Jill! You can't just walk away from that!" For the first time in my life I heard true honor being offered to me. I could discern it, and I believed that I could trust it.

A few days after returning to Arlington, Kirk called and invited me to his family's cabin in New Mexico. He offered to fly me to Amarillo and drive me to Angel Fire to meet up with his parents and sister. I had not seen them in over twenty years, and it would be like seeing long-lost relatives. I could hardly say no, but I told him I would think about it. Laura said she'd kill me if I didn't go. Still, I pictured it to be like a private high school reunion. Kirk and I would hold hands on some mountaintop, like Forrest Gump and Jenny, and then finally go our separate ways.

God is providential. He sent the worst snowstorm to hit that part of New Mexico in thirty years. Before ever leaving

Amarillo, Kirk and I got snowed in for four days with his sister and brother-in-law. They secretly prayed for us nonstop throughout those four days. I watched Kirk's heart as he interacted with his older sister. They are the best of friends. I remembered who he was.

Then, he did this silly little move that he does with his arms in the air, and I instantly, accidentally fell flat on my face in love with him again. I remembered those arms. If there was one significantly healing thing about Kirk when we dated in high school, it was the way his arms made me feel. He was tall, skinny, and a little wiry back then. His arms felt as if they'd wrap around me two or three times, and I would hide my face from life inside that affection. I find it amazing and so sweet that the Lord specifically said, "He will be my arms." After praying and praying and more praying, we met with each other's pastors to pray with them and seek their advice. With their initially cautious, yet soon contented approval, we were married two months later and moving to sunny California. I do not know how the Lord could have brought me any closer to physical virginity than to lead me into this merciful covenant marriage with my first love.

My mother offered to buy the wedding dress. The experience will remain one of my most cherished moments with her. We stood in a bridal shop together and I watched her eyes light up as she stepped up to it. She seemed to almost glow as she gently extended the shear, pearl-colored beaded sleeves to get a better look. She had picked out the most beautiful, fairytale-worthy, *white* wedding dress for me.

Each of us is a broken person in the never-ending process of restoration and daily renewal. We are making our way through the delicate dynamics of this life together. Every step of the way I have been swept off my feet by God's amazing grace and mercy for such undeserving people.

Kirk and I now stand side by side with our hands in the air, in praise, for the victory we've found in Him. We love Him and will worship Him forever. Ephesians 3:20-21 says, "Now unto Him that is able to do exceeding abundantly above all that we ask or think, according to the power that worketh in us, unto Him be the glory in the church and in Christ Jesus unto all generations for ever and ever. Amen" (KJV).

The...new beginning.